Ear Disease
A Clinical Guide

Michael Hawke, MD
Department of Otolaryngology
University of Toronto
Toronto, ON

2003
Decker DTC
Hamilton • London

Decker DTC
An Imprint of BC Decker Inc
P.O. Box 620, L.C.D. 1
Hamilton, Ontario L8N 3K7
Tel: 905-522-7017; 800-568-7281
Fax: 905-522-7839; 888-311-4987
E-mail: info@bcdecker.com
www.bcdecker.com

© 2003 Michael Hawke, MD

All rights reserved. Without limiting the rights under copyright reserved above, no part of this publication may be reproduced, stored in or introduced into a retrieval system, or transmitted, in any form or by any means (electronic, mechanical, photocopying, recording, or otherwise), without the prior written permission of the publisher.

03 04 05 06/FP/9 8 7 6 5 4 3 2 1

ISBN 1-55009-241-3

Printed in Canada

Sales and Distribution

United States
BC Decker Inc
P.O. Box 785
Lewiston, NY 14092-0785
Tel: 905-522-7017;
 800-568-7281
Fax: 905-522-7839;
 888-311-4987
E-mail: info@bcdecker.com
www.bcdecker.com

Canada
BC Decker Inc
20 Hughson Street South
P.O. Box 620, LCD 1
Hamilton, Ontario L8N 3K7
Tel: 905-522-7017;
 800-568-7281
Fax: 905-522-7839;
 888-311-4987
E-mail: info@bcdecker.com
www.bcdecker.com

Foreign Rights
John Scott & Company
International Publishers' Agency
P.O. Box 878
Kimberton, PA 19442
Tel: 610-827-1640
Fax: 610-827-1671
E-mail: jsco@voicenet.com

Japan
Igaku-Shoin Ltd.
Foreign Publications Department
3-24-17 Hongo
Bunkyo-ku, Tokyo, Japan 113-8719
Tel: 3 3817 5680
Fax: 3 3815 6776
E-mail: fd@igaku-shoin.co.jp

U.K., Europe, Scandinavia, Middle East
Elsevier Science
Customer Service Department
Foots Cray High Street
Sidcup, Kent
DA14 5HP, UK
Tel: 44 (0) 208 308 5760
Fax: 44 (0) 181 308 5702
E-mail: cservice@harcourt.com

Singapore, Malaysia, Thailand, Philippines, Indonesia, Vietnam, Pacific Rim, Korea
Elsevier Science Asia
583 Orchard Road
#09/01, Forum
Singapore 238884
Tel: 65-737-3593
Fax: 65-753-2145

Australia, New Zealand
Elsevier Science Australia
Customer Service Department
STM Division
Locked Bag 16
St. Peters, New South Wales, 2044
Australia
Tel: 61 02 9517-8999
Fax: 61 02 9517-2249
E-mail: stmp@harcourt.com.au
www.harcourt.com.au

Mexico and Central America
ETM SA de CV
Calle de Tula 59
Colonia Condesa
06140 Mexico DF, Mexico
Tel: 52-5-5553-6657
Fax: 52-5-5211-8468
E-mail: editoresdetextosmex
@prodigy.net.mx

Argentina
CLM (Cuspide Libros Medicos)
Av. Córdoba 2067 - (1120)
Buenos Aires, Argentina
Tel: (5411) 4961-0042/(5411) 4964-0848
Fax: (5411) 4963-7988
E-mail: clm@cuspide.com

Brazil
Tecmedd
Av. Maurílio Biagi, 2850
City Ribeirão Preto – SP –
CEP: 14021-000
Tel: 0800 992236
Fax: (16) 3993-9000
E-mail: tecmedd@tecmedd.com.br

Notice: The authors and publisher have made every effort to ensure that the patient care recommended herein, including choice of drugs and drug dosages, is in accord with the accepted standard and practice at the time of publication. However, since research and regulation constantly change clinical standards, the reader is urged to check the product information sheet included in the package of each drug, which includes recommended doses, warnings, and contraindications. This is particularly important with new or infrequently used drugs. Any treatment regimen, particularly one involving medication, involves inherent risk that must be weighed on a case-by-case basis against the benefits anticipated. The reader is cautioned that the purpose of this book is to inform and enlighten; the information contained herein is not intended as, and should not be employed as, a substitute for individual diagnosis and treatment.

CONTENTS

Acknowledgments iv

Chapter 1
  Diseases of the Pinna 1

Chapter 2
  Diseases of the External Auditory Canal 26

Chapter 3
  Diseases of the Tympanic Membrane
  and Middle Ear 54

Index 89

Dedication

For Nikki and Ellie

Acknowledgments

This pocket guide would not have been possible without the vision and support of the Ear Nose and Throat Division of Alcon. Particular thanks are due to Chuck Inman, Group Product Director, Global Otic, whose commitment to excellence and education was responsible for this project.

These otoscopic photographs would not have been possible without the generous support and technical assistance provided by Karl Storz.

Thanks are also due to my publisher, Rochelle Decker of BC Decker Inc, who has made this project a delight. It was Rochelle's idea to include a companion CD of images that can be used by the reader for educational purposes.

Michael Hawke, MD

Chapter 1

DISEASES OF THE PINNA

Figure 1–1

Normal pinna. In the human, the pinna plays a rudimentary function in the amplification and localization of sound, in addition to providing protection by shielding the external canal from direct trauma. Because the pinna is attached to the side of the head in a relatively exposed position, it is traumatized easily.

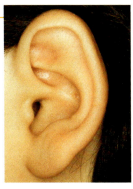

Figure 1–2

The auricular cartilage. The shape of the pinna is determined by the underlying auricular cartilage. The auricular cartilage of the pinna is contiguous with the cartilage of the outer (cartilaginous) portion of the external auditory canal.

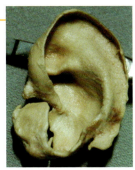

CONGENITAL MALFORMATIONS OF THE EAR

Figure 1–3

Darwin's tubercle. Darwin's tubercle is a small cartilaginous protuberance that is most commonly located along the concave edge of the posterosuperior margin of the helix and projects anteriorly. Darwin's tubercles are inherited by means of an autosomal dominant gene that has a variable expressivity. This atavistic remnant represents the apex of the anthropoid ear, suggesting a common ancestry between humanity and apes, and for this reason it is called "Darwin's" tubercle.

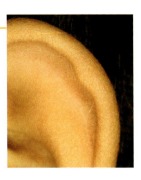

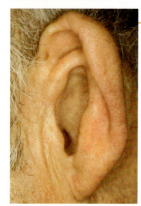

FIGURE 1–4

Partial meatal atresia. Absence or partial maldevelopment of the pinna is frequently associated with abnormalities of the external auditory canal and underlying middle ear; the inner ear in these patients is usually normal. In the case shown here, the anterior half of the conchal bowl is not fully developed, giving the ear a feline appearance. The external canal consists of only a small conchal pit that ends blindly a short distance medially. This failure in the development of the external auditory meatus is associated with deformity of the middle ear and ossicles.

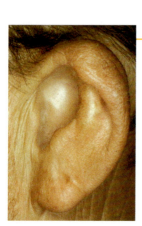

FIGURE 1–5

Complete meatal atresia. In this patient, there is no opening for the external canal (complete meatal atresia).

FIGURE 1-6

Microtia. The term "microtia" is used when there is gross hypoplasia of the pinna with a blind or absent external auditory canal. Microtia encompasses a wide spectrum of severe malformations, ranging from a mere nubbin of tissue with no recognizable features on the side of the head to an incompletely formed auricular appendage. Microtia is typically bilateral, although the degree of the deformity may be different on the two sides. Children born with microtia should have their hearing tested soon after birth and, if hearing loss is present, be fitted with a hearing aid as quickly as possible.

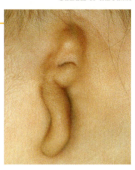

FIGURE 1-7

Outstanding ears (posterior view). Outstanding, or protruding ears are the most common cosmetic deformity of the pinna. They are inherited by means of an autosomal dominant gene that has complete penetrance but a variable expressivity. Although outstanding ears are asymptomatic, children with such ears often experience intense emotional discomfort, and otoplasty is recommended for cosmetic reasons.

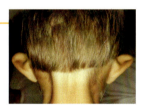

FIGURE 1-8

Outstanding ears (posterior view). The angle between the auricle and the side of the head is greater than normal, and the auricle protrudes anteriorly.

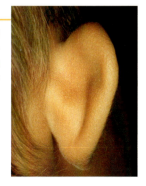

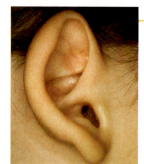

Figure 1–9

Outstanding ears (lateral view). There may be a poorly formed antihelical fold or excessive tissue, usually in the conchal or triangular fossae, giving the ear a cupped appearance.

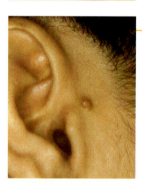

Figure 1–10

Preauricular tag. Preauricular tags are tiny, raised nubbins of skin located along the anterior border of the ear in front of the tragus. They are soft, mobile, and filled with soft tissue.

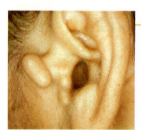

Figure 1–11

Accessory auricle. The pinna is formed in the embryo by the coalescence of six tiny hillocks, or tubercles, located on the dorsal end of the first (mandibular) and second (hyoid) branchial arches. Accessory auricles represent the remnant of one of the embryologic hillocks. They differ from preauricular tags in that they contain a small island of cartilage. Preauricular tags and accessory auricles are often excised for cosmetic reasons.

Figure 1-12

Preauricular pit. Defective closure of the first branchial cleft or a failure in the fusion of the primitive ear hillocks may result in the formation of a small pit, sinus, or fistula in front of the pinna. These deformities can vary from a small dimple (preauricular pit) to a larger sinus (preauricular sinus). Preauricular pits are shallow invaginations in the skin of the face located just in front of the anterior border of the anterior crus of the helix. A foul-smelling, cheesy discharge of desquamated keratin debris is often encountered.

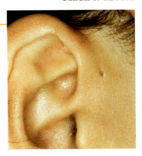

Figure 1-13

Infected preauricular sinus. A preauricular sinus is deeper than a pit and is lined with a stratified, squamous, keratinizing epithelium. Gentle sounding with a small lacrimal duct probe can be used to establish the depth of the preauricular depression and distinguish a preauricular pit from a preauricular sinus. Preauricular pits and sinuses can become infected, and if they do, the infection frequently recurs.

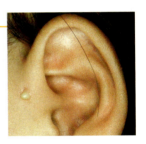

Figure 1-14

Preauricular cyst. If the opening of a preauricular sinus becomes occluded, the sinus will be converted into a cyst. As the keratin squames of the skin lining the interior of the cyst shed into its lumen, the cyst will slowly enlarge. Preauricular sinuses and cysts may be closely related to the facial nerve, and for this reason, their removal should be left to an experienced surgeon.

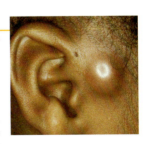

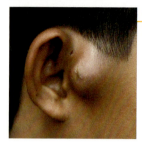

Figure 1–15

Infected preauricular sinus. If pathogenic bacteria enter the opening of a preauricular sinus, the tract may become infected. When the tract of an infected preauricular sinus is patent, a milky, purulent material will be seen oozing onto the surface of the skin (see Figure 1–13). When the opening of the preauricular sinus is occluded, then an abscess may form. Pain, tenderness, and swelling in front of the anterior border of the helix suggests the presence of a preauricular abscess. Once a preauricular sinus has become infected, there is a strong likelihood of recurrent infection.

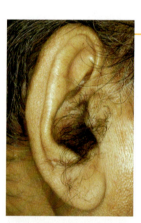

Figure 1–16

Hairy tragus. With age, coarse hairs appear on the tragus of some males. This is a secondary sexual characteristic that is called a "hairy tragus."

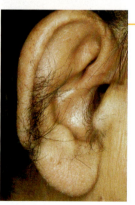

Figure 1–17

Hairy pinna. Coarse hairs may appear on the lower portions of the helix of some individuals as they age. This type of ear is referred to as a "hairy pinna". Hairy pinna occurs only in men and is a Y chromosome-linked trait.

Figure 1–18

Hypertrichosis lanuginosa acquisita. Hypertrichosis lanuginosa acquisita is an acquired condition characterized by the excessive growth of fine, villous hair. It has been associated with certain metabolic conditions (porphyria) and some medications (minoxidil).

Reproduced with the permission of Dr. M.A. Knowling and the Editor of the *Canadian Medical Association Journal*

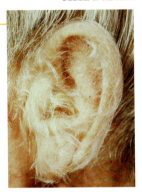

Figure 1–19

Idiopathic cystic chondromalacia (auricular pseudocyst). Benign idiopathic cystic chondromalacia is an idiopathic cystic degeneration of the auricular cartilage that presents clinically as an isolated, unilateral, asymptomatic, cystic swelling of the pinna. Aspiration produces a clear, uninfected, yellow, serous fluid.

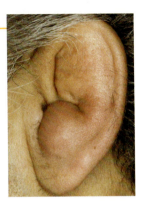

Figure 1–20

Traumatic seroma. Acute or chronic friction that irritates the perichondrium of the auricular cartilage can induce a subperichondrial serous or serosanguinous effusion. A seroma should be aseptically aspirated to prevent devitalization and subsequent necrosis of the underlying cartilage.

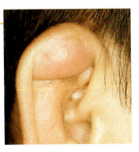

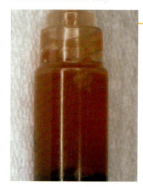

Figure 1–21

Aspirate from a traumatic seroma. Note the clear serosanguinous aspirate. After the fluid has been aspirated, the perichondrium should be gently compressed onto the cartilage by an inert (stainless steel or monofilament nylon) mattress suture using a button on either side of the pinna to maintain gentle pressure for 10 to 14 days to prevent reaccumulation of the fluid.

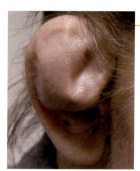

Figure 1–22

Large subperichondrial hematoma. Hematomas of the auricle are usually the result of blunt trauma, such as those encountered during boxing, rugby, and other physical activities in which the skin of the pinna is exposed to twisting or shearing forces. The small blood vessels that lie between the perichondrium and the underlying auricular cartilage are easily ruptured by a shearing force. Once a vessel is torn, blood will leak into the subperichondrial plane (between the perichondrium and the cartilage), thereby elevating the perichondrium from the underlying cartilage. The subperichondrial hematoma shown here has formed a fluctuant purple bulge that balloons the skin over the lateral surface of the pinna and distorts its normal sharp contours.

FIGURE 1–23

Small subperichondrial hematoma. If the subperichondrial collection of blood is not removed, it will deprive the underlying cartilage of its critical nourishment, thereby producing an avascular necrosis of the involved cartilage. Simple aspiration of the hematoma is not sufficient, as it will almost always recur. A late sequela is the organization of the hematoma by the ingrowth of fibrous tissue and the development of a cauliflower ear.

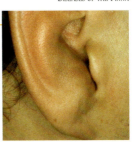

FIGURE 1–24

Small subperichondrial hematoma post-drainage. The entire collection of blood should be aspirated under sterile conditions and the skin held down against the underlying cartilage by mattress sutures. Antibiotic coverage should be provided to prevent the development of acute perichondritis and subsequent cartilage necrosis.

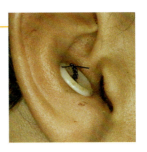

FIGURE 1–25

Cauliflower ear. Repeated episodes of blunt trauma to the pinna (eg, after boxing, rugby, or football) can produce areas of subperichondrial separation or hemorrhage, which will cause necrosis and softening of the underlying auricular cartilage. The fibrosis that develops during the healing of these damaged areas usually results in both thickening and deformity of the lateral surface of the pinna. This type of post-traumatic deformity is called a "cauliflower ear."

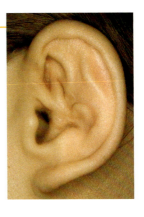

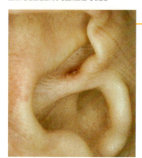

Figure 1–26

Ear mold pressure ulceration. Chronic pressure on the skin by a poorly fitting hearing-aid ear mold can cause a traumatic pressure ulcer.

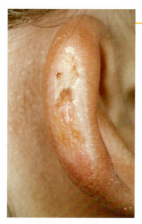

Figure 1–27

Solar dermatitis (sunburn). Because of its exposed location, the superior portion of the pinna is exposed to the sun and therefore is highly susceptible to acute solar dermatitis (sunburn). Repeated exposure of the skin to solar radiation predisposes an individual to premaligant and malignant cutaneous changes.

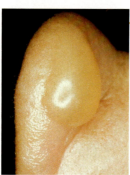

Figure 1–28

Frostbite. The pinna, by virtue of its exposed location, presents a large surface area in relation to its blood supply and is consequently subject to damage from extreme cold. Exposure to very low temperatures causes a severe and prolonged vasoconstriction of the capillary walls, resulting in damage to these walls. The anesthesia that takes place in those areas of the skin exposed to the cold allows a significant amount of damage to occur "silently" without the individual's knowledge.

The upper third of the pinna is most commonly affected by frostbite. Frostbite is usually characterized by a reddish or blue discoloration of the pinna, often accompanied by serum-filled blisters that resemble a second-degree burn.

FIGURE 1–29

Late calcification of the auricular cartilage following frostbite. Delayed dystrophic calcification of the underlying auricular cartilage may develop years after the initial frostbite. When this occurs, the pinna is bony and hard to palpation. A radiograph of the pinna will reveal radiodense areas of calcification in the auricular cartilage.

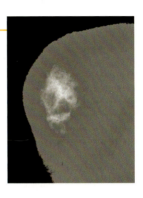

FIGURE 1–30

Early herpes zoster (shingles). Herpes zoster is an acute localized cutaneous infection of a sensory dermatome by the *Varicella zoster* virus. It first appears as a series of pustules.

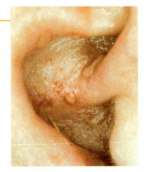

FIGURE 1–31

Late herpes zoster (shingles). Over time, the pustules rupture, and the lesions crust.

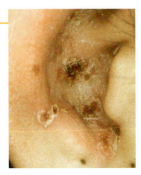

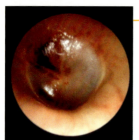

Figure 1-32

Herpes zoster of the tympanic membrane. Herpes zoster oticus is characterized by the appearance of vesicles on the skin of the pinna in the region of the conchal bowl, along the skin of the external auditory canal, and, occasionally, on the tympanic membrane.

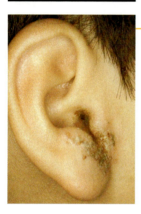

Figure 1-33

Impetigo. The superficial layers of the epidermis may become infected with *Staphylococcus aureus* or *Streptococcus pyogenes*. Macerated and moist skin is particularly susceptible to bacterial infections. The initial lesion consists of an infected vesicle or pustule that ruptures and dries to produce typical yellowish crusts. Both the pustules and the crusts contain viable bacteria and are highly contagious.

Impetigo is surprisingly painless, and the most common symptom is the presence of crusty scabs and local itching. Treatment consists of the application of a topical cream containing an antibiotic that is effective against the causative organisms.

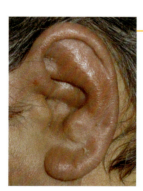

Figure 1-34

Acute perichondritis. Acute perichondritis of the auricle is a bacterial infection of the perichondrium and underlying cartilage that develops usually following trauma to the skin of the pinna. A painful, red, and swollen pinna following localized infection of the external ear, trauma, or surgery suggests the development of an acute perichondritis.

This type of acute bacterial infection is potentially serious because, if untreated, the underlying auricular cartilage will become infected and, ultimately, necrotic, with collapse of the pinna. Gram-negative bacteria, especially *Pseudomonas aeruginosa* and *Proteus*, are the usual causative organisms.

Figure 1–35

Relapsing perichondritis. Relapsing perichondritis is an autoimmune episodic recurrent inflammation of the cartilaginous structures of the body. Clinically, relapsing perichondritis is characterized by recurrent, always bilateral, auricular, nasal, and laryngeal chondritis. These patients have antibodies to Type II collagen.

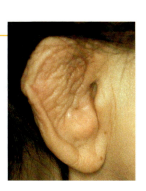

Reproduced courtesy of Dr. Benjamin Fisher.

Figure 1–36

Erysipelas. Erysipelas is an acute, rapidly spreading, superficial cellulitis caused by group A β-hemolytic *Streptococcus*. It is characterized by a bright red, tender swelling that is well demarcated from the surrounding normal skin.

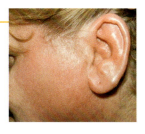

Figure 1–37

Creased lobule. The appearance of a crease running across the skin of the lobule is a minor deformity that does not appear until later life. Most commonly, the crease begins where the ear lobe attaches to the head and angles diagonally downwards and backwards to the edge of the lobule. This sign is associated with increasing age and also, independently, with an increased incidence of obstructive coronary artery disease.

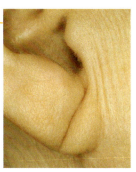

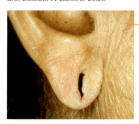

Figure 1-38

Elongated earring hole. Over time, the continued wearing of a heavy earring may gradually elongate an earring hole.

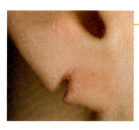

Figure 1-39

Split lobule. If an earring is pulled through the lobule and the defect is not sutured, the lobule will remain split (bifid). These injuries usually occur when a large earring is accidentally grasped and pulled by an infant or child.

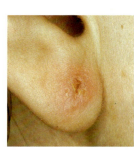

Figure 1-40

Infected earring tract. Localized infection within the epithelial-lined fistula tract of a pierced ear is usually the result of poor hygiene. There will be localized tenderness, erythema, swelling, and, occasionally, crusting. Pressure on the lobule will frequently expel a tiny drop of pus.

This type of infection can usually be avoided by good personal hygiene. If the infection does not respond to topical antibiotic therapy, the earring may need to be removed.

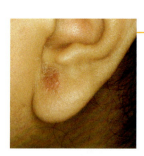

Figure 1-41

Contact dermatitis. Contact dermatitis of the external ear is relatively common and can frequently be confused with infectious dermatitis. One important differentiating feature is that patients with contact dermatitis complain primarily of itching rather than pain. Another important diagnostic clue is a track-like extension of the allergic inflammatory response below the ear as the discharge carries the allergen along.

The offending allergen may be a topical medication, such as neomycin, or one of the ingredients of topical ear drops, an ear mold, or an earring. Treatment consists of avoiding the offending allergen and applying a mild steroid-containing topical cream to the involved areas.

FIGURE 1–42

Metal contact dermatitis of the lobule. Cutaneous allergy (contact dermatitis) to metals, especially to nickel, may develop when the gold plating covering a poor-quality earring wears off and the underlying metal comes into direct contact with the underlying skin of the lobule. A localized area of contact dermatitis is frequently seen under an earring.

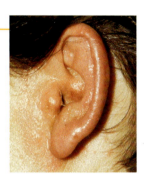

FIGURE 1–43

Hypertrophic scars. A simple hypertrophic scar should be differentiated from a keloid (Figure 1–44). Hypertrophic scars remain within the confines of the wound and flatten spontaneously over 1 or more years. In contrast, keloids persist and extend beyond the site of the original injury.

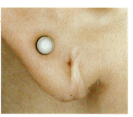

FIGURE 1–44

Keloids. Keloids are the result of an abnormality in a wound's healing process in which excessive bulk is produced at the site of a cutaneous injury, most commonly following a laceration, a surgical incision around the ear, or ear piercing. Keloids occur more commonly in blacks than in whites and develop most frequently in the second and third decades of life. In the case shown here, the keloid developed following ear piercing.

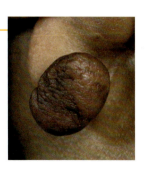

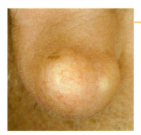

Figure 1–45

Post-traumatic epidermal inclusion cyst. Fragments of cutaneous epithelium can become trapped in the dermis of the lobule following ear piercing. If this happens, an epidermoid cyst will develop from the entrapped remnants.

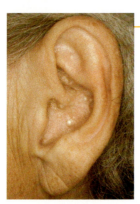

Figure 1–46

Milia. Milia are small, multiple, white, keratin-filled cysts that arise from the infundibulum in the region of the sebaceous duct. Milia differ from epidermal cysts only in size.

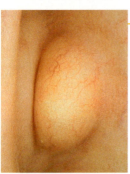

Figure 1–47

Epidermal cysts. Epidermal cysts are slow-growing, round, firm, intradermal cysts that arise most commonly from the infundibula of hair follicles. The most common sites for the development of epidermal cysts are along the postauricular sulcus and the medial aspect of the lobule at its junction with the face.

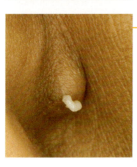

Figure 1–48

Epidermal cyst showing cheesy debris. Clinically, these cysts appear as smooth, round, doughy masses that may have a tiny surface opening. The overlying skin is frequently yellowish-white because of the mass of pure white keratin contained within the cyst. Note the cheesy debris that is being expressed from this cyst.

Figure 1–49

Infected epidermal cyst. If an epidermal cyst becomes infected, the lining of the cyst may rupture, and the keratin squames within the cyst can spill out into the surrounding soft tissue.

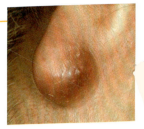

Figure 1–50

Drainage of an infected epidermal cyst. An acute foreign body granulomatous reaction can develop in response to the keratin squames that infiltrate the tissue surrounding an infected epidermal cyst. Clinically, this can give rise to local tenderness. An incision into the cyst for drainage may be required, as seen here.

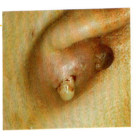

Figure 1–51

Neurodermatitis. Itching is the common feature in chronic infective dermatitis and may provoke the patient into repeated scratching of the involved area. The term "neurodermatitis" is used when the chronic dermatitis appears to be the result of trauma from repeated scratching,

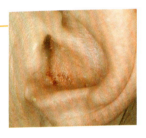

The infecting organisms may be bacterial (most commonly *Staphylococcus aureus* or *Streptococcus*), fungal (most commonly *Candida albicans*), or, not infrequently, a mixture of both. These superficial infections respond well to topical antibiotic and/or antifungal therapy combined with good hygiene.

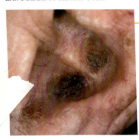

Figure 1-52

Neglect keratosis. In the elderly, neglected areas of skin may accumulated keratin debris over time. These raised, greasy, pigmented "lesions" resemble seborrheic keratosis at first glance. The diagnosis is, however, readily established, however, because these areas of neglect keratosis are easily removed by friction to reveal normal underlying skin.

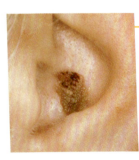

Figure 1-53

Seborrheic Keratosis. Seborrheic keratoses are benign, cutaneous tumors that appear as distinct, raised, pigmented, greasy lesions. The lesions appear to be "stuck on" to the surface of the skin, but a close examination of the surface of the keratosis will reveal keratotic plugs filling irregular crypts. Seborrheic keratoses vary in color from light yellow through brown to black.

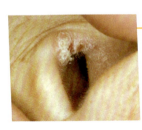

Figure 1-54

Psoriasis. Psoriasis is a hereditary disorder of the skin that is characterized by an increased rate of epidermal cell replication. The chronic relapsing dermatosis shown here is characterized by sharply defined, dry, erythematous patches covered with adherent, silvery white scales. If the scales are removed by gentle scraping, fine, punctate bleeding points may be seen (the Ausspitz sign). When psoriasis involves the external ear, the patient may also have typical lesions on the auricle.

Figure 1-55

Psoriasis of the external canal. Psoriasis may involve the external ear and the entrance to the external canal. The ear canal may be occluded by a toothpaste-like accumulation of desquamative keratin debris. If psoriasis is suspected in an otherwise asymptomatic patient with persistent accumulation of debris in the canal, the elbows and the scalp should be inspected, as these are the most common sites for psoriasis.

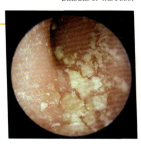

Figure 1-56

Gouty tophus. In advanced cases of gout, a collection of uric acid crystals may appear on the helix as a tophus. Gouty tophi present as painful, skin-covered nodules that occur most commonly on the helix. On palpation, the nodule is gritty, and yellow, crystal-like structures can occasionally be seen through the skin. Today, with modern medical treatment, gouty tophi are rarely encountered.

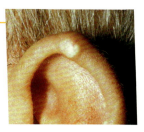

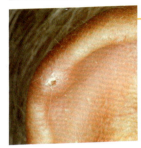

Figure 1-57

Chondrodermatitis nodularis helicus chronica (Winkler's nodule). Chondrodermatitis nodularis helicus chronica is a discrete, firm, raised, and frequently tender, or even painful, nodule usually located on the apex of the helix of the ear. This lesion occurs primarily in middle-aged and elderly males, and is the result of solar damage to the skin covering the top of the pinna with resulting late solar elastosis. Repeated minor trauma and poor blood supply to the helical rim are responsible for degeneration of the skin, the underlying dermis, and the auricular cartilage. A central epidermal channel or pit (which develops for the purpose of transepidermal extrusion of the degenerated dermal collagen) is commonly seen.

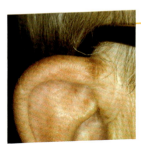

Figure 1-58

Solar lentigo. Solar lentigines are multiple, brown, flat, irregular, uniformly pigmented cutaneous lesions that develop in skin that has been repeatedly exposed to the sun.

Figure 1-59

Solar keratosis. Solar keratoses are lesions, considered to be premalignant, that arise on areas of the skin that have been repeatedly exposed to the sun. These lesions occur most commonly in fair-skinned individuals after the third decade of life. Clinically, solar keratoses appear as dry, rough, adherent, and scaly lesions. Although a solar keratosis can develop over time into a squamous cell carcinoma, the tumor that develops is usually less malignant than the usual squamous cell carcinoma, which arises de novo.

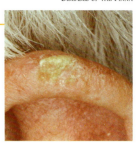

Figure 1-60

Cutaneous horn (solar keratosis). Occasionally, solar keratoses produce a circumscribed, conical, hyperkeratotic excrescence, which is termed a "cutaneous horn." Because solar keratoses are premalignant, they should be excised.

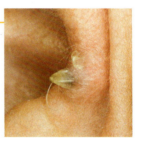

Figure 1-61

Pigmented nevus. Pigmented lesions occur frequently on the external ear. The presence of an enlarging or darkly pigmented lesion should always arouse the examiner's suspicion that this may, in fact, represent a malignant melanoma. The lesion shown here is a benign pigmented nevus.

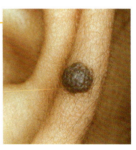

Figure 1-62

Verruca vulgaris. Verruca vulgaris (wart) is a benign localized area of epithelial hyperplasia caused by the human papilloma virus. Clinically, a verruca appears as a circumscribed, elevated papilloma that has a filiform or papillomatous hyperkeratotic surface.

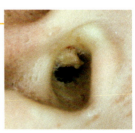

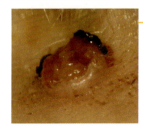

FIGURE 1-63

Keratoacanthoma. Keratoacanthomas are benign, usually solitary, rapidly developing epithelial neoplasms that arise most frequently on the sun-exposed areas of fair-skinned, elderly individuals. The lesion consists of a firm, dome-shaped nodule that has skin-colored, rolled edges and a central crater filled with keratin debris. A keratoacanthomas usually begins as an erythematous papule that enlarges rapidly over 2 to 8 weeks to reach a maximum size of 1 to 2 cm; if left alone, it will involute spontaneously within 6 to 12 months, leaving behind a puckered and often unsightly scar.

Unfortunately, keratoacanthomas resemble squamous cell carcinomas both clinically and histologically. When the diagnosis is in doubt, and to avoid the scarring that accompanies spontaneous involution, an excisional biopsy is usually indicated.

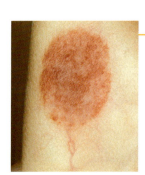

FIGURE 1-64

Capillary hemangioma. A capillary hemangioma (strawberry birthmark) is a flat, bright red, soft, benign tumor consisting of numerous small, blood-filled capillaries. Most capillary hemangiomas resolve spontaneously during the first decade of life.

Figure 1-65

Arteriovenous malformation. An arteriovenous malformation presents as discoloration and distortion of the skin overlying the pinna. Palpation will reveal pulsations and auscultation an audible bruit.

Reproduced courtesy of Dr. David P. Mitchell.

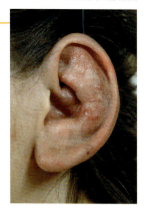

Figure 1-66

Basal cell carcinoma. The presence of persistent ulceration of the external ear should suggest the possibility of a malignancy. The patient shown here had been treated for many months for a chronic infection of the external ear when, in fact, she had an extensive basal cell carcinoma involving the conchal bowl. The diagnosis was established by biopsy. Fortunately, the tumor responded to radiotherapy.

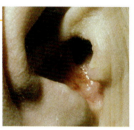

Figure 1-67

Basal cell carcinoma. More commonly, the proliferation of basal cells creates a raised, indurated nodule with firm, pearly edges. A small central crust is frequently present, underneath which is a central ulcer.

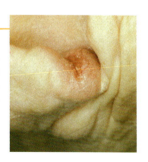

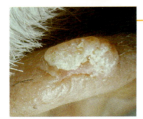

Figure 1-68

Verrucous carcinoma. Verrucous carcinoma is a low-grade exophytic slowly growing squamous cell carcinoma that is wart-like in appearance.

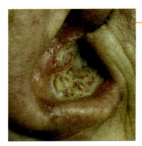

Figure 1-69

Squamous cell carcinoma. Squamous cell carcinoma of the auricle occurs most frequently in persons of fair complexion who have experienced long exposure to sunlight. Clinically, a squamous cell carcinoma may appear as an indurated papule, plaque, or nodule that is frequently eroded, crusted, and ulcerated. Rapid growth in the size of the lesion, tenderness to palpation, crusting, and ulceration are all signs that should alert the physician to the presence of squamous cell carcinoma. On palpation, the lesion is hard and may be fixed to the underlying structures. There may also be spread to the regional lymph nodes.

Congenital abnormalities of the ear can be unilateral or bilateral and, of course, may be associated with congenital malformations elsewhere in the body. These deformities may be the result of a genetic defect, viral infection, or exposure to ototoxic drugs during the first trimester of pregnancy.

Severe congenital malformations of the pinna are often associated with an abnormality of the underlying middle or inner ear. As the external, middle, and inner ears differ in both their embryological origins and times of development, there is a wide variation in the types of abnormality that can be encountered.

Patients may be seen who have an absent auricle and external auditory canal and yet have only a minimal deformity of the middle ear and a normal inner ear. By contrast, some children have a normal or almost normal external ear but a severe congenital malformation of the underlying middle and inner ears.

A CT scan should be obtained to determine if the middle ear structures are sufficiently normal for middle ear reconstructive surgery to be successful.

Definitive treatment requires a complete excision of the entire sinus tract. Great care must be taken during the excision of a preauricular sinus because the sinus may extend quite deeply and be closely related to the branches of the facial nerve.Rarely, a preauricular fistula will be found as an abnormal communication between the skin of the face or neck and the external auditory canal (collaural fistula).

Preauricular sinuses are usually asymptomatic unless they become infected.

CHRONIC INFECTIVE DERMATITIS

Healthy skin usually provides an effective physical and chemical barrier against the numerous bacteria and fungi present in our environment. Under conditions of repeated trauma, moisture or maceration, the skin loses this effective barrier. The result may be an acute or chronic superficial infection of the epidermis by bacteria, fungi, or a mixture of both organisms.If the infection does not respond to the initial topical medication, a culture of the involved area should be taken for both bacteria and fungi and the medication adjusted accordingly. If the infection still does not respond, a biopsy may be needed to establish a diagnosis.

Chapter 2

DISEASES OF THE EXTERNAL AUDITORY CANAL

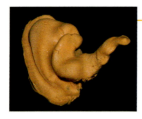

Figure 2-1

The external auditory canal. The external auditory canal (EAC) is a skin-lined canal that connects the tympanic membrane to the exterior via the conchal bowl. The EAC is divided into two distinct portions: the outer "cartilaginous" canal and the inner "bony" auditory canal.

The tortuous shape of the canal and its relationship to the pinna can be seen in this postmortem impression.

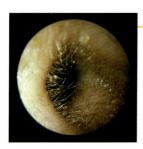

Figure 2-2

The cartilaginous external auditory canal. The outer third of the EAC is surrounded by cartilage. The surrounding cartilaginous framework allows the cartilaginous canal a moderate amount of mobility. The skin lining the cartilaginous canal is **thick** and contains numerous appendages (hairs, ceruminous glands, sebaceous glands, and sweat glands).

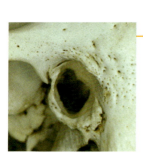

Figure 2-3

The tympanic bone. The inner two-thirds of the external auditory canal is surrounded by the tympanic bone.

Figure 2-4

The bony portion of the EAC. The skin lining the bony canal is thin and has no appendages. Because this **thin** skin is closely adherent to the underlying tympanic bone, it is both immobile and easily traumatized.

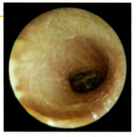

Figure 2-5

Normal epithelial migration. The epithelium covering the surface of the tympanic membrane and external auditory canal possesses a unique self-cleansing mechanism. The outermost superficial layers of corneocytes of the skin in this area desquamate by migrating radially **off** the surface of the tympanic membrane and then **laterally** along the bony canal to the outer cartilaginous canal, where the superficial keratin squames are shed into the ceruminous material.

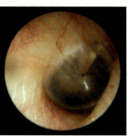

Figure 2-6

Ink dot at 2 months. Epithelial migration, which accounts for the normal self-cleansing properties of the ear canal, can be observed by following, over a period of weeks, the path of a dot of India ink that has been applied to the surface of the tympanic membrane (see Figure 2-5). Two months later, the ink dot has migrated in a radial direction to a position overlying the area of the incudostapedial joint.

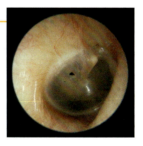

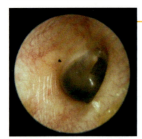

Figure 2-7

Ink dot at 4 months. By 4 months, the dot has migrated laterally onto the bony external auditory canal.

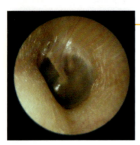

Figure 2-8

The tympanic membrane. The tympanic membrane is a pale gray, semi-transparent membrane, positioned obliquely at the medial end of the external auditory canal. The tympanic membrane is formed of three layers: an outer epithelial layer, which is continuous with the skin of the bony external auditory canal; a fibrous supporting middle layer, which gives the tympanic membrane its strength and shape; and an inner mucosal layer, which is continuous with the mucosal lining of the tympanic cavity.

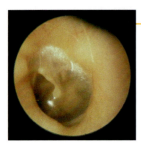

Figure 2-9

The pars tensa. The lower four-fifths of the tympanic membrane contain a well-organized, fibrous middle layer called the "pars tensa." The handle of the malleus, which is embedded in the pars tensa, can be seen extending downwards and backwards, ending at the apex of the "triangular cone" of reflected light. The long process of the incus and its articulation with the head of the stapes can frequently be seen through the posterosuperior quadrant of a thin normal tympanic membrane.

Figure 2-10

The pars flaccida (Shrapnell's membrane) and the chorda tympani. **The upper fifth of the tympanic membrane, the "pars flaccida" (Shrapnell's membrane) has a sparser, less well-organized middle layer than the pars tensa and is more mobile.** The chorda tympani nerve, which supplies taste to the anterior two-thirds of the tongue, is sometimes visible behind the posterosuperior quadrant of the tympanic membrane, passing horizontally across the middle ear between the long process of the incus and the handle of the malleus.

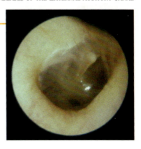

Figure 2-11

The vascular strip. The surface of the tympanic membrane receives its blood supply from the deep auricular branch of the maxillary artery. Branches of this artery can frequently be seen as a visible leash of blood vessels that run down the superior canal wall. This area is called the "vascular strip."

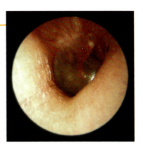

Figure 2-12

Keratin patches. If a normal tympanic membrane is examined carefully, multiple discrete, thickened, whitish patches can be seen on its surface. These patches consist of tiny stacks of keratinocytes that have developed as the superficial layers of keratin split apart during their normal outward migration. Maceration of the outer surface of the tympanic membrane by moisture or edema of the tympanic membrane (eg, during acute otitis media) enhances the visibility of these keratin patches.

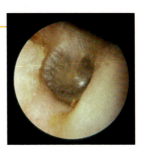

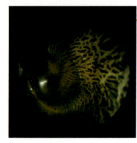

Figure 2-13

Keratin patches demonstrated by osmium staining (cadaveric specimen). The shape and distribution of keratin patches can be demonstrated clearly by staining the surface of a cadaveric tympanic membrane with a solution of 1% osmium tetroxide. The osmium stain is taken up by the keratin patches, dying them black.

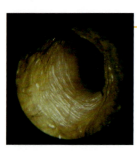

Figure 2-14

Transverse wrinkles of the deep canal. Transverse wrinkles are surface corrugations or waves that lie at right angles to the long axis of the external canal. These wrinkles develop as the normal outwardly migrating superficial layer of the stratum corneum of the deep canal becomes heaped up against the stationary adnexal structures, especially the hairs of the superficial canal. Transverse wrinkles are present in most deep canals, where they are most readily visible on the posterior surface.

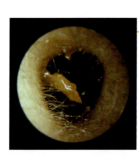

Figure 2-15

Normal cerumen. The ceruminous glands are modified sweat glands located in the outer cartilaginous canal. These glands produce a clear, colorless secretion that is properly called "cerumen." In most individuals, the secretions of the ceruminous glands and the outwardly migrating keratin squames continue to migrate laterally and are spontaneously discharged from the external canal by the normal process of migration.

Figure 2-16

Veil of cerumen. In some individuals, a thin "veil" of cerumen will be seen draped across the lumen of the EAC. These patients will complain of hearing loss if the veil completely seals off the canal. Such a veil is usually the result of the insertion of a cotton-tipped applicator that has elevated and rotated the superficial layer of outwardly migrating keratin.

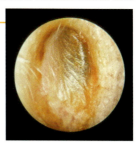

Figure 2-17

The colors of cerumen. Normal cerumen varies in color from a light golden yellow through brown to black.

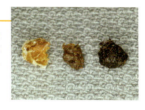

Figure 2-18

The "true" color of cerumen. The pigment responsible for the color of cerumen has yet to be identified. The "true" color of cerumen appears to be burnt ocher, as demonstrated in this smear made from a piece of dark brown cerumen.

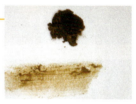

Figure 2-19

Cerumen accumulation. The ear canal is often occluded by cerumen (earwax), which must be removed if the entire tympanic membrane is to be seen and a proper otoscopic examination accomplished. Although cerumen is normally removed from the external canal by the process of epithelial migration, in some patients, there is a failure of migration, which results in cerumen accumulation within the canal.

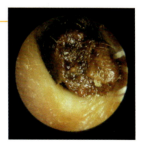

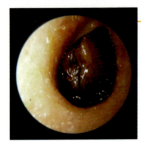

Figure 2-20

Wet cerumen. Cerumen (earwax) is an accumulation of secretions from the ceruminous glands, mixed with keratin desquamated from the skin of the external canal. Cerumen has two consistencies: wet cerumen and dry cerumen. Wet (soft) cerumen is moist, sticky, and usually brown. The keratin contained within a wet cerumen plug consists of small sheets of keratin squames.

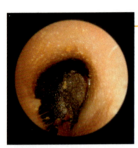

Figure 2-21

Dry cerumen. In contrast, dry cerumen is hard, dry, and usually dark brown or black. The keratin contained within dry cerumen consists of large, densely compacted sheets of keratin squames.

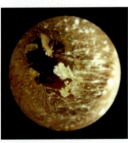

Figure 2-22

"Oriental" cerumen. Cerumen in many Asians is different from that in non-Asians. These individuals have cerumen that is dry, golden yellow, and extremely flaky. In Asia, this type of earwax is referred to as "rice bran" wax.

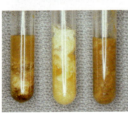

Figure 2-23

Effective cerumenolytics. Cerumenolytics are compounds that soften and loosen earwax. The only truly effective cerumenolytics are aqueous. Note the swelling and dissolution of the plugs of hard dry cerumen caused by three different aqueous solutions. From the left: distilled water, hydrogen peroxide, and sodium bicarbonate.

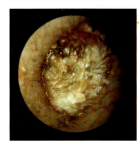

Figure 2-34

Keratosis obturans. Although the precise etiology of keratosis obturans remains unclear, it appears that there is an increased rate of desquamation of corneocytes within the deep canal combined with a failure of the normal outward migration of these epithelial cells from the surface of the tympanic membrane laterally along the surface of the skin lining the external canal. The result is the accumulation of keratin squames within the external canal. The bony meatus is occluded by a plug of compressed, pearly white keratin debris.

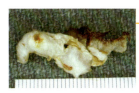

Figure 2-35

Plug of keratin debris. This white mass of compressed keratin squames was removed from the external canal of the patient shown in Figure 2-34.

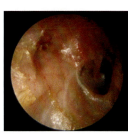

Figure 2-36

Keratosis obturans: widened deep external canal. Over time, as the plug of accumulating keratin squames continues to enlarge, it exerts pressure on the walls of the deep meatus, gradually stimulating resorption of the bony walls of the surrounding canal. This is seen clinically as widening of the deep meatus. After removal of the plug of compressed keratin squames, hyperemia of the underlying canal skin and superficial granulations arising from the underlying inflamed skin are frequently seen.

Figure 2-30

Fresh blood clot. Any clot in the meatus should be removed carefully so that the deeper structures can be examined.

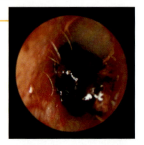

Figure 2-31

Inspissated old blood clot. It is much easier to remove a fresh, soft, jelly-like clot before it turns into a stony, hard, black, tar-like mass, as seen here.

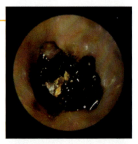

Figure 2-32

Keratin foreign-body granuloma. Most lacerations of the external ear canal heal completely without visible scarring. Occasionally, a keratin foreign-body granuloma develops, caused by the implantation of keratin squames into the dermis. In these cases, exuberant granulation tissue at the site of the laceration forms 1 or 2 weeks after the injury. Removal of the granulation tissue and the implanted foreign material (superficial corneocytes) is usually required to allow healing.

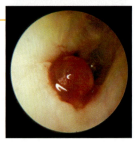

Figure 2-33

Epidermal inclusion cyst. A small epithelial inclusion cyst may develop if epithelial cells have been trapped in the dermis. These tiny cysts appear as a pearly white, round swelling in the skin of the external canal. Epidemal inclusion cysts rarely enlarge.

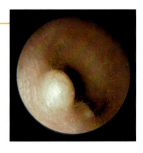

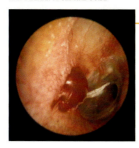

Figure 2-27

Large external-canal hematoma. Larger hematomas elevate the skin of the canal, appearing as a red bleb. With time, the bright red color darkens, and the subepidermal collection of blood is resorbed. Although no treatment is required, a discussion of the danger of inserting objects into the deep external auditory canal is advisable.

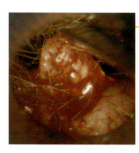

Figure 2-28

External-canal laceration. Although the skin of the bony canal is extremely thin and easily traumatized, it is protected from external trauma by its deep location. Most lacerations occur in the skin of the more accessible cartilaginous canal. In the case shown here, a flap of skin has been raised. These lacerations are usually the result of inadvertent self-manipulation by the patient.

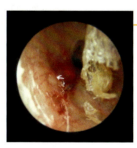

Figure 2-29

Actively bleeding laceration. The ear should be examined carefully to ensure that the laceration is confined to the canal skin and does not involve the tympanic membrane or middle ear. In those cases where the laceration is the result of a head injury, the possibility of a fracture of the skull base should be considered.

The bleeding from a laceration is generally self-limiting. The ear should be kept dry to avoid possible infection. Where the laceration may have been contaminated, the use of a suitable topical antibiotic ear drop is recommended.

Figure 2-24

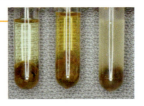

Ineffective cerumenolytics. Organic solutions may lubricate a cerumen plug; however, they are ineffective in breaking up cerumen, as demonstrated in these three samples. From the left: olive oil, Cerumenex,™ and Cerumol.™

Figure 2-25

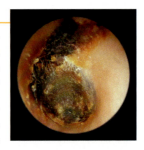

Cotton swab abuse. Individuals who frequently use cotton swabs to clean their ears often push their cerumen back into the deep meatus until it lies directly against the tympanic membrane. In these circumstances, loosening of the cerumen with an effective cerumenolytic prior to syringing is advisable.

Figure 2-26

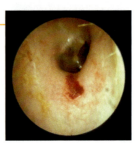

Small external-canal hematoma. A hematoma of the skin of the external auditory canal is usually the result of direct physical trauma to the thin and delicate skin of the deep (bony) external canal from an object (eg, matchstick or cotton-tipped applicator) that has been inserted into the ear canal. Hematomas are usually asymptomatic and indicate that the skin of the ear canal has recently been traumatized. **A small hematoma will appear as a bright red linear streak along the skin of the deep canal.**

FIGURE 2-37

Keratosis obturans: automastoidectomy. In rare cases, the bony erosion caused by the gradually enlarging keratin plug is so extensive that an automastoidectomy is carried out. Great care must be taken in removing the plug because the erosion might have resorbed the bone overlying the facial nerve in its vertical portion and that over the jugular bulb.

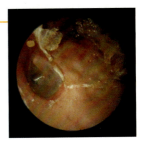

KERATOSIS OBTURANS TREATMENT GUIDELINES

The aim of treatment is, first, to remove the keratin plug safely and completely and, second, to prevent recurrence. Any inflammation of the ear canal skin or secondary otitis externa should be treated with a suitable topical antibiotic ear drop. As this idiopathic condition has a tendency to recur, these patients should be seen in follow-up on a regular basis, so that any accumulation of keratin can be removed before the lumen of the canal becomes totally obstructed.

FIGURE 2-38

Benign osteitis of the external ear canal. Benign osteitis of the tympanic bone appears to result from a traumatic laceration and subsequent ulceration of the skin of the deep meatus. This ulceration results in necrosis of the underlying periosteum, with exposure, infection (osteitis), and, ultimately, devitalization and sequestration of the underlying tympanic bone. Fresh granulations and an accumulation of white keratin debris may be found covering the base of the ulcer.

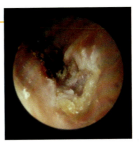

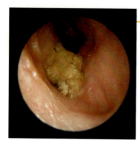

Figure 2-39

Benign osteitis of the external ear canal. The typical ulceration in the skin covering the floor of the deep meatus may not be seen until the ear canal has been cleaned and the area over the exposed tympanic bone debrided. Following cleansing and debridement of the base of the ulcer, exposed, abnormally yellowish tympanic bone will always be found. The clinical course of this disease is relatively mild, and, over time, spontaneous sequestration of the dead bone and reepithelialization of the ulcer will occur.

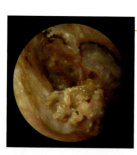

Figure 2-40

Irradiation osteitis. Therapeutic radiation may cause osteoradionecrosis of the tympanic bone with ulceration and, ultimately, sequestration of the necrotic tympanic bone. The clinical appearance and course of irradiation osteitis are similar to that described previously for benign osteitis of the tympanic bone.

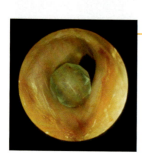

Figure 2-41

Foreign body: plastic bead. A wide variety of foreign bodies have been discovered in the external auditory canal. The symptoms will depend on the nature of the foreign body. Relatively inert materials may produce no symptoms and be discovered only inadvertently during a routine otoscopic examination, whereas organic material tends to cause a localized external otitis.

Figure 2-42

Foreign body: foam rubber. The type of foreign body present can usually be recognized without difficulty. The aim is to remove the foreign body as safely and expeditiously as possible while avoiding damage to the delicate skin of the deep external auditory canal, the tympanic membrane, and the middle ear.

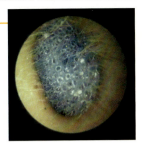

Figure 2-43

Foreign body: large pebble. The method of removal depends on the type of foreign body present. If the tympanic membrane is intact, then gentle syringing is generally both safe and effective.

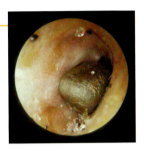

Figure 2-44

Foreign Body: cockroach. Occasionally the fluttering or scratching movements of a living insect will cause considerable distress.

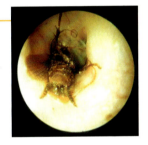

Figure 2-45

Foreign body: Schuknecht foreign body remover. Smooth, hard, round objects such as beads are best removed with a funnel-shaped Schuknecht suction tip foreign body remover.

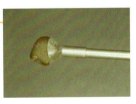

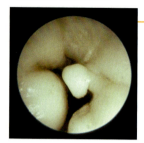

Figure 2-46

Exostoses arising from the tympanic bone (temporal bone specimen). Exostoses arise in susceptible individuals in response to the repeated stimulation of the bony external canal by cold water. Exostoses appear as round or oval, hard, smooth, discrete excrescences, which are sometimes pedunculated and may be single or multiple.

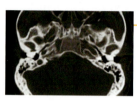

Figure 2-47

Exostoses: CT scan. The initial cold-induced vasoconstriction of the deep canal is followed by a reactive hyperemia and stimulation of the periosteum lining the medial surface of the tympanic bone, which lays down consecutive layers of dense subperiosteal bone. The dense ivory bone of an exostosis is readily seen in a CT scan.

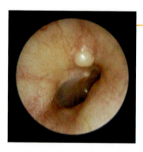

Figure 2-48

Small solitary exostosis. Note the small solitary exostosis arising from the tympanic bone just above the head of the malleus. The skin overlying the exostosis is usually thinner and paler than normal. A single exostosis can be differentiated from a foreign body or cyst by gentle palpation with a blunt probe.

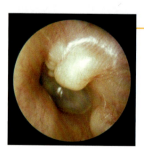

Figure 2-49

Large solitary exostosis. Over time, with repeated exposure to cold water, an exostosis will continue to enlarge. If the patient prevents further entry of cold water into the ear canal by wearing earplugs, then the exostosis will not enlarge.

Figure 2-50

Multiple exostoses. Note the multiple exostoses, which obscure most of the tympanic membrane. Because most exostoses are asymptomatic, they usually require no treatment.

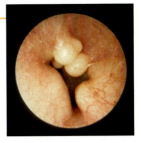

Figure 2-51

Exostoses blocking the canal. Exostoses are usually asymptomatic unless they become large enough to cause a hearing loss by blocking the external canal or entrap cerumen.

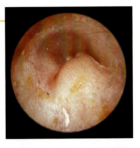

Figure 2-52

Osteoma of the external canal. Osteomas of the external canal are true benign bony tumors. They are usually solitary, appearing as a bony, hard, sessile mass covered by normal canal skin. The "bony" nature of these tumors can be determined by palpation. Unlike exostoses, osteomas frequently trap wax and keratin debris in the deep meatus, producing a conductive hearing loss. If an osteoma produces symptoms by occluding the lumen of the canal or by trapping wax and keratin debris within the canal, it should be removed surgically.

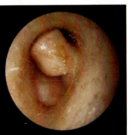

OTITIS EXTERNA

Healthy skin usually provides an effective physical and chemical barrier against the numerous bacteria and fungi present in our environment. Under conditions of repeated trauma, moisture, or maceration, the skin loses this effective barrier. The result may be an acute or chronic superficial infection of the epidermis by bacteria, fungi, or a mixture of both organisms. Most cases of chronic otitis externa are self-inflicted, due to repeated contamination of the ear with water and/or self-manipulation. The education in the principles and importance of good aural hygiene is an essential component of the treatment of otitis externa.

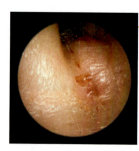

Figure 2-53

Furuncle (acute circumscribed otitis externa). A furuncle is a staphylococcal abscess arising from the base of a hair follicle. Furuncles result from the entry of pyogenic staphylococci into the skin of the superficial external canal. They occur only in the outer cartilaginous portion of the external canal, as the skin of the bony canal is hairless. Because the skin of the external canal is adherent to the underlying perichondrium, even a small furuncle will produce severe local pain, which is aggravated by movement of the pinna, pressure on the tragus, or chewing.

If the furuncle is obviously pointing, it can be punctured with a large sterile hypodermic needle, bringing relief from pain. The patient is usually seen at an early stage, however, when incision is of little value. Suitable analgesics and a full course of an oral broad-spectrum antibiotic effective against *Staphylococcus* is indicated.

Figure 2-54

Early acute diffuse otitis externa (swimmer's ear). Acute diffuse otitis externa (swimmer's ear) is an acute, diffuse, painful bacterial infection of the skin of the external auditory canal. The chief agents responsible for the development of acute diffuse otitis externa are local trauma and moisture. Gram-negative bacteria, principally *Pseudomonas aeruginosa*, can be cultured in most cases. The skin of the external canal is swollen, extremely tender, and shiny. Severe pain is usually present.

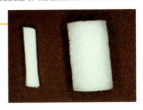

Figure 2-55

Severe acute diffuse otitis externa. A *peau d'orange* ("orange skin") appearance is occasionally seen and is due to lymphedema. When the lumen of the meatus is obliterated, it is usually impossible to examine the tympanic membrane. In severe cases, the ear may be so tender that even the gentlest movement of the pinna will cause excruciating pain, and the introduction of the smallest speculum available will be resisted by the patient. The most commonly prescribed topical ear drops contain an antibiotic effective against Pseudomonas, eg, ciprofloxacin, together with a corticosteroid to reduce inflammation. The attending physician should ascertain that the tympanic membrane is intact when prescribing any topical antibiotic drop that contains potentially ototoxic substances (eg, gentamycin) to ensure that the ototoxic material cannot enter the middle ear and come into contact with the inner ear via the round window membrane or the oval window.

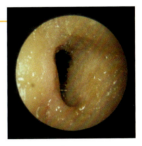

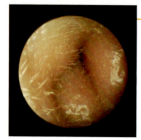

FIGURE 2-56

Pope Otowick. If local treatment is to be effective, the canal must be cleaned thoroughly after a swab has been taken for bacterial and fungal cultures. For topical therapy to be effective, the medication must be able to make direct contact with the underlying skin of the canal. When the lumen of the canal has been narrowed by edema, the patient will be unable to instill the topical preparation into the occluded ear canal, and a Pope Otowick should be gently eased as far as possible into the canal, moistened, and then impregnated with a suitable topical antibiotic and antiinflammatory preparation.

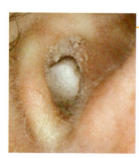

FIGURE 2-57

Pope Otowick inserted in an occluded ear canal (severe acute otitis externa). The wick should be replaced on a daily basis until the edema has subsided and the topical drops can be instilled directly into the canal. In the extremely severe case, the simultaneous administration of oral ciprofloxacin and a short course of high-dose prednisone may be beneficial. Appropriate analgesics and hypnotics are also indicated when acute otitis externa causes severe pain.

OTOTOXICITY WARNING

Ototopical antibiotics are often prescribed for individuals with acute and chronic otitis externa, infected ventilation tubes, acute and chronic otitis media with tympanic membrane perforation, and/or infected mastoid cavities.

All aminoglycoside-containing ear drops carry potential risk for ototoxicity (both cochlear and vestibular) if they reach the middle ear through a defect in the tympanic membrane. Although it is impossible to assess the actual incidence of topical aminoglycoside ototoxicity (possibly estimated at 1/10,000), it is not negligible and is probably more common than once thought.

Adverse Drug Reaction (ADR) warnings have been previously issued by Health Canada concerning aminoglycoside ear drops and ototoxicity (CMAJ 1997;156(7):1056-8) in this regard.

A recent study by Bath and colleagues (Laryngoscope 1999;109: 1088-93) has demonstrated that inadvertent toxicity appeared to occur when topical drops were typically used for longer than 7 days. The toxicity from topical gentamicin appeared to be primarily vestibular, not cochlear.

In the presence of a temporomandibular (TM) perforation, the following precautions should be taken into account when topical aminoglycoside drops are prescribed:

1. The drops should be used for the shortest duration possible and **never** in the presence of what amounts to a normal, healthy-looking middle ear.

2. The patient should be instructed precisely regarding the duration and dosage of therapy and advised to stop treatment as soon as the discharge stops.

3. Therapy should not exceed 5 to 7 days without a reassessment.

4. The patient should be advised to stop treatment immediately if hearing loss, tinnitus, vertigo, or imbalance is noted.

5. When otorrhea persists despite an appropriate trial of medical treatment, referral to an ear, nose and throat (ENT) specialist should be considered.

6. Finally, in all patients with tympanic membrane defects, the risks of using aminoglycoside otic preparations should be carefully weighed against the potential benefits.

7. The prescribing physician must document the above in the patient record.

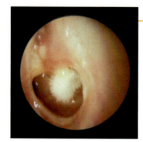

Figure 2-58

Otomycosis: aspergillus in the middle ear. Fungi may cause either acute or chronic otitis externa. *Aspergillus niger, A. flavus, A. fumigatus,* and *Candida albicans*, are the organisms most commonly encountered. Predisposing factors include moisture (eg, swimming or showering) and the previous use of topical antibiotic ear drops, especially those containing neomycin, which may kill off the normal flora of the external canal. Symptoms of otomycosis include itching, local irritation, persistent otorrhea, and severe pain.

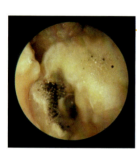

Figure 2-59

Acute aspergillus otitis externa. In the early stages, examination generally reveals a cotton wool-like appearance or debris that resembles moist tissue paper. In advanced cases, the ear canal may be filled with a whitish or creamy, thick material. There may be a fluffy appearance due to the presence of a mass of tiny mycelia (see Figure 2-58). When the infection is caused by *Aspergillus niger*, it may be possible to identify the tiny, grayish-black conidiophores (fruiting heads), as seen here.

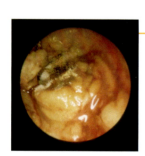

Figure 2-60

Severe acute aspergillus otitis externa. In severe infections, with ulceration of the canal skin, blood and purulent material will fill the external canal. Thorough aural toilet by suction or gentle syringing to remove all of the debris is the cornerstone of effective treatment. An appropriate topical antifungal preparation is then applied.

FIGURE 2-61

Severe acute aspergillus otitis externa. The underlying canal skin and tympanic membrane is often inflamed and ulcerated because of invasion by fungal mycelia. Refractory cases may require repeated aural toilet, with reapplication of the antifungal agent.

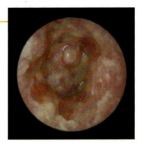

FIGURE 2-62

Chronic candidal otitis externa. In many patients, the typical appearance of the fungus is masked by debris, and the correct diagnosis can be reached only by sending a sample of the material for fungal culture. This is particularly true for Candida albicans, which has no specific visual diagnostic features.

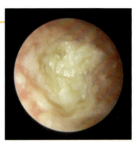

FIGURE 2-63

Chronic otitis externa with keratin debris. Chronic otitis externa is usually the result of poor aural hygiene. Itching is the common feature in chronic infective dermatitis and may provoke the patient into repeated scratching of the involved area. The otoscopic appearances in chronic otitis externa are variable. Normal epithelial desquamation and migration are impaired, and moist keratin debris will frequently accumulate within the lumen of the external canal.

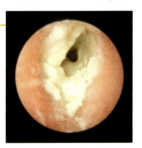

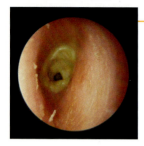

Figure 2-64

Chronic otitis externa with purulent exudates. A foul-smelling, thick, purulent exudate may be found within the meatus. The first step is to send a swab for bacterial and fungal culture to identify the causative organisms and assist in the selection of the appropriate topical antibiotic or antimycotic agent. All debris from the ear canal must be removed if topical therapy is to be successful.

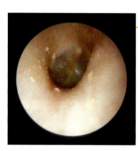

Figure 2-65

Chronic otitis externa from chronic cotton bud abuse. In those patients who are compulsive "ear cleaners," the only signs of chronic otitis externa may be a slight redness of the epithelium and the absence of cerumen or debris, as shown here. The mainstay of treatment is the modification of those behaviors that have contributed to the development of the disease, eg, scratching, compulsive cleansing, and repeated exposure of the ear to moisture.

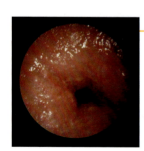

Figure 2-66

Acute allergic otitis externa: neomycin contact dermatitis. In refractory cases of acute and chronic otitis externa, the examiner should be on the look-out for allergic reactions to the medications used, eg, neomycin contact dermatitis. The possibility of an underlying dermatologic disorder, systemic disease, or even malignancy must always be considered in unresponsive cases.

FIGURE 2-67

Moderate acquired external-canal stenosis. Canal stenosis may develop as the result of trauma to the skin of the external auditory canal. The trauma may be the result of an accidental laceration, chronic self-manipulation, or chronic otitis. Once the skin lining the external canal has been lacerated, exuberant granulations within the external canal can epithelialize, producing a skin-covered fibrous-tissue stenosis. The stenosis occurs most commonly in the narrowest portion of the external canal (the isthmus).

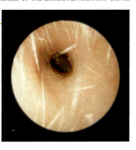

FIGURE 2-68

Severe acquired external-canal stenosis. If the stenosis is wide, it will allow migration of the epithelium from the deep canal to the outside to occur normally. In severe cases, the lumen may be reduced to a tiny pinhole, behind which desquamated keratin may become trapped.

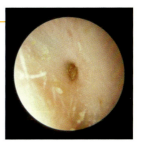

Figure 2-69

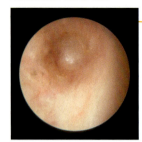

False fundus. A false fundus is an acquired condition in which the external auditory canal ends blindly at the bony cartilaginous junction. A false fundus can develop following an extremely severe injury to the epithelial lining of the external ear canal if granulation tissue is produced at the isthmus in such quantity that it totally occludes the ear canal and then becomes epithelialized. A false fundus is usually recognized when the medial end of the external canal ***is closer*** to the speculum during otoscopic examination than the examiner would normally anticipate. A false fundus lacks the normal anatomical landmarks of the tympanic membrane. It has an abnormal thickness resembling skin, as compared to the translucency of a normal tympanic membrane.

FIGURE 2-70

Necrotizing otitis externa (malignant otitis externa). Necrotizing otitis externa is a severe, aggressive, invasive form of otitis externa that occurs in elderly diabetics and otherwise immunocompromised patients. Necrotizing otitis externa is potentially lethal from the fulminating spread of infection, which may involve the temporal bone, the cranial nerves, and the cranial contents. The causative organism is usually Pseudomonas aeruginosa. The initial symptoms are those of an acute otitis externa, with local pain and discharge from the ear canal. The first step towards the correct diagnosis is ***clinical suspicion*** (ie, ***severe otitis externa in a diabetic or immunocompromised individual***). As the infection progresses, the pain becomes severe and unremitting, and cranial nerve palsy deficits may appear. A hallmark of malignant otitis externa is an area of infected granulation tissue on the floor of the cartilaginous ear canal near the junction between the cartilaginous and bony portions of the canal.

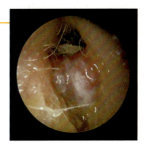

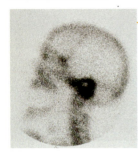

Figure 2-71

Malignant otitis externa: gallium 67 scan. It is critical that necrotizing otitis externa be diagnosed at an early stage so that appropriate treatment can be initiated before the osteomyelitis has spread beyond the possibility of treatment. Necrotizing otitis externa is characterized by the progressive spread of infection from the ear canal into the adjacent structures. The infection may spread into the temporal bone, causing osteomyelitis, or extend to the base of the skull, resulting in multiple cranial nerve palsies, meningitis, brain abscess, or death. A gallium 67 citrate bone scan will reveal the infected focus in the involved temporal bone by binding to the granulocytes.

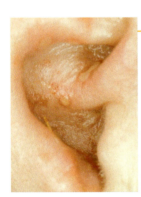

Figure 2-72

Herpes zoster oticus (Ramsay Hunt syndrome). Herpes zoster oticus is a viral infection of the geniculate ganglion (seventh cranial nerve), characterized by a vesicular eruption of the skin of the external ear. Herpes zoster oticus may also be associated with a herpes infection of the upper cervical roots or the glossopharyngeal nerve, the latter producing vesicles on the soft palate. Initially, the patient experiences a hot feeling within the ear, which rapidly develops into pain of increasing severity. Hearing loss, tinnitus, or vertigo may be present when the inner ear is involved and facial paralysis if the facial nerve is involved. Note the characteristic vesicles on the conchal bowl.

Figure 2-73

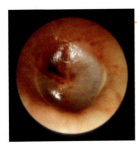

Herpes zoster oticus: tympanic membrane. Vesicles may also appear along the skin of the external canal and sometimes even on the tympanic membrane. The patient should be started immediately on a course of oral acyclovir. Topical acyclovir ointment can be applied to the cutaneous lesions. The vesicles should be kept dry and an oral antipruritic administered to prevent scratching and subsequent secondary infection.

Figure 2-74

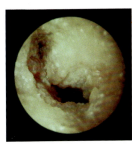

Squamous cell carcinoma. No otoscopic signs are truly diagnostic of malignant tumors of the external auditory canal. The most suspicious symptoms are ***bleeding*** from the external canal and chronic otorrhoea that has recently become associated with ***pain***. ***When pain or bleeding develops*** in cases of chronic otitis externa or chronic suppurative otitis media, a careful inspection of the ear must be carried out to exclude the possibility of an underlying neoplasm. Any unusual or uncharacteristic growths arising in the external canal must have a biopsy.

CHAPTER 3

DISEASES OF THE TYMPANIC MEMBRANE AND MIDDLE EAR

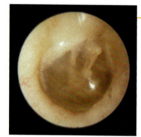

FIGURE 3–1

The normal tympanic membrane.
The normal tympanic membrane is a pale gray, oval, semitransparent membrane set obliquely at the medial end of the bony external auditory canal. The triangular "cone of light" is a reflection back down the canal of light from the otoscope by the only portion of the tympanic membrane that is at right angles to the central axis of the external auditory canal.

A portion of the most lateral ossicle, the handle of the malleus, is visible extending downwards and backwards, with a flattened end (the umbo) that sits at the apex of the cone of light. The lateral process of the malleus is a small, white protuberance arising from the upper end of the handle of the malleus.

The long process of the incus, including its articulation with the head of the stapes, and the chorda tympani nerve passing between the handle of the malleus and the long process of the incus can frequently be seen through a thin tympanic membrane.

Figure 3-2

The apparent shape of the tympanic membrane. The tympanic membrane is actually circular; however, because it is positioned at an oblique angle to the central axis of the external ear canal, it appears to the examiner as an oval disk.

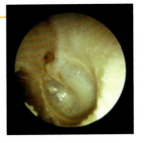

Figure 3-3

The true shape of the tympanic membrane. The true circular shape of the tympanic membrane can be seen in this photograph of the eardrum shown in Figure 3.2, which was taken through a hole drilled in the mastoid at right angles to the surface of the tympanic membrane.

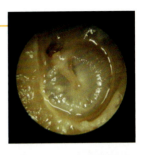

Figure 3-4

Congenital epidermal inclusion cyst of the tympanic membrane. The small, white, round cyst arising from the lateral surface of the tympanic membrane is a congenital epidermal inclusion cyst. These benign cysts are located lateral to the fibrous middle layer of the eardrum.

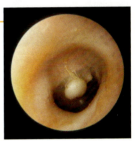

Figure 3-5

Traumatic tympanic membrane perforation. Traumatic perforations of the tympanic membrane are caused two mechanisms: **violent changes in the air pressure** within the external auditory canal and middle ear (eg, from a slap on the ear or as the result of an explosion) or **direct physical trauma** to the tympanic membrane (eg, the insertion of cotton-tipped applicators, bobby pins, or matchsticks).

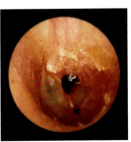

Sudden pressure changes within the external canal usually produce perforations of the anteroinferior quadrant. The large anteroinferior perforation shown here was caused by a slap on the ear. A small hematoma is seen underneath the handle of the malleus. This type of perforation characteristically has everted, ragged edges because the initial positive pressure wave is followed by a high negative wave that sucks the margins of the perforation laterally.

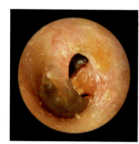

Figure 3–6

Healing traumatic tympanic membrane perforation. One month later, the perforation shown in Figure 3–5 has healed, and the scab under which the healing occurred has been carried off the tympanic membrane onto the skin of the bony canal by the normal migratory process. Ossicular damage is uncommon in this type of perforation; however, the effects of the violent pressure change on the cochlea can cause a sensorineural hearing loss.

In those pressure-change perforations that are caused by the detonation of an explosive device ("blast perforations"), the implosive force, in addition to perforating the tympanic membrane, can in some cases be conducted through the perilymph, producing a rupture of the round window membrane This results in a leakage of perilymph into the middle ear and produces a sudden and often severe sensorineural hearing loss, with or without associated vertigo and nystagmus. If the rupture remains patent (a perilymph fistula), the sensorineural hearing loss can fluctuate.

FIGURE 3–7

Direct-trauma tympanic membrane perforation. Perforations that result from the insertion of foreign materials into the ear canal (direct trauma) usually occur posteriorly because this is the most directly accessible portion of the tympanic membrane. The edges of the perforation can be hemorrhagic, and fresh blood may be seen in the deep meatus. The perforation seen in the posterosuperior quadrant of the tympanic membrane shown here occurred when a cotton-tipped applicator was inserted too deeply into the ear canal.

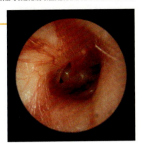

FIGURE 3–8

Healed direct-trauma tympanic membrane perforation. Six weeks later, the perforation has healed with no visible scarring. Most small and medium-sized traumatic perforations heal spontaneously within 3 months. Perforations that do not heal may require surgical closure.

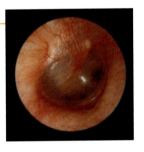

Direct-trauma perforations are frequently associated with ossicular damage, because both the incus and its articulation with the stapes are located directly behind the posterosuperior quadrant of the tympanic membrane.

FIGURE 3–9

Middle ear barotrauma (barotraumatic otitis media). Otitic barotrauma occurs when the atmospheric pressure is significantly higher than the pressure within the middle ear cleft and eustachian tube function is inadequate, eg, during descent in an aircraft or diving in water.

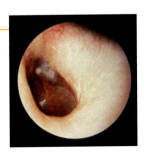

The otoscopic appearances of otitic barotrauma are variable and include erythema of the tympanic membrane; solitary or multiple interstitial hemorrhages of the tympanic membrane, often with streaking in patches in the pars flaccida and along the sides of the handle of the malleus; a golden-yellow serous exudate (see below); or even a frank hemotympanum.

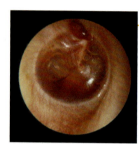

Figure 3–10

Middle ear barotrauma showing serous exudate. The symptoms of barotraumas are variable and include stuffiness, ear pain, and hearing loss. The presence of serous fluid within the middle ear can produce a "swishing" sensation, brought about by head movement. The effects of established barotrauma usually resolve spontaneously within 6 weeks.

Individuals can usually prevent otitic barotrauma by avoiding air travel when upper respiratory tract infections are present. If this is impossible, the use of a topical nasal decongestant drop such as xylometazoline hydrochloride 0.1% and oral systemic decongestants, combined with regular autoinflation by the Valsalva maneuver during descent, are helpful.

Figure 3-11

Hemotympanum. A hemotympanum (the presence of extravasated blood or blood-stained fluid in the middle ear) can develop following barotrauma, epistaxis, head injury, or a temporal bone fracture.

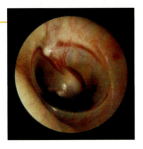

In the classic hemotympanum, the middle ear fills with blood, and the tympanic membrane appears uniformly bright red, dark red, brown, or gun metal blue, depending on the color of the bloody fluid within the middle ear.

Figure 3-12

Aspirate from a hemotympanum. The aspirate from a hemotympanum consists of red, dark blue, or brown fluid. The treatment of a hemotympanum is essentially that of the underlying cause. The hemotympanum will usually resolve spontaneously. If resolution does not occur, however, the fluid can be drained through a myringotomy.

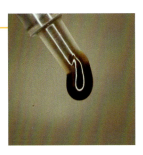

Figure 3-13

"Chocolate Eardrum." In long-standing cases of hemotympanum, degradation of the hemoglobin occurs, and the dark brown coloration is referred to as a "chocolate eardrums."

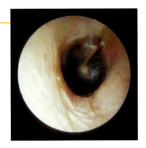

Figure 3–14

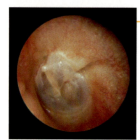

Temporal bone fracture. A head injury can result in a fracture of the temporal bone. Longitudinal fractures of the temporal bone (the most common) frequently run through the roof of the middle ear (the tegmen tympani), causing a hemotympanum. Less common is rupture of the tympanic membrane, with resultant bleeding into the external canal. The bony annulus may be fractured. Backwards displacement of the condyle of the mandible from a blow to the chin can cause a fracture of the anterior wall of the bony external canal. If a watery discharge persists, the possibility of a cerebrospinal-fluid leak (CSF otorrhea) should be considered.

The telltale sign of a temporal bone fracture is a deformity of the annulus or bony canal wall resulting from the displaced fragments of bone. Temporal bone fractures heal by fibrous union, and long after the original injury, the telltale sign of a fracture line might still be visible otoscopically, usually on the posterosuperior canal wall near the annulus.

Figure 3–15

Bullous myringitis (myringitis bullosa). Bullous myringitis is a distinctive form of otitis externa, characterized by the appearance of fluid-filled hemorrhagic blebs on the tympanic membrane and skin of the deep external meatus. Severe local pain within the ear is usually the first symptom and is usually followed by the spontaneous appearance of a blood-tinged serous or serosanguineous discharge. Although the agent responsible for bullous myringitis has not been identified conclusively, both influenza viruses and *Mycoplasma pneumoniae* are suspect.

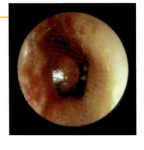

The tympanic membrane is covered by multiple blebs (blisters) filled with either a serous (shown here) or a serosanguineous fluid (Figure 3–16). Petechial hemorrhages are commonly seen in the skin around the base of the blebs.

Figure 3–16

Bullous myringitis showing blebs filled with serosanguineous fluid. A conductive hearing loss can result from the development of a secondary serous otitis media. Because there is no specific treatment for the causative organism, therapy is directed towards adequate analgesia and the prevention of secondary infection by keeping the ear clean and dry.

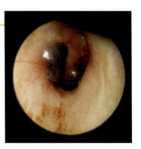

In rare cases, inner ear involvement with sensorineural hearing loss and vertigo can occur.

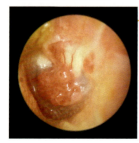

FIGURE 3–17

Granular myringitis. Granular myringitis is a chronic inflammation of the external surface of the tympanic membrane (myringitis) associated with an ulceration of the outer epithelial layer of the tympanic membrane and the production of exophytic granulation tissue. Otoscopically, localized areas of bright red granulation tissue are seen arising from the lateral surface of the tympanic membrane. Painless mucopurulent otorrhea is the most common symptom.

A swab of any discharge within the canal should be sent for bacterial and fungal culture to identify pathogens present within the canal. Granular myringitis can be an extremely difficult condition to treat. If the appropriate topical steroid-containing antibacterial or antifungal preparations do not produce resolution, then surgical removal of the granulations might be necessary.

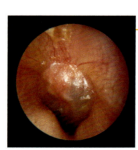

FIGURE 3–18

Acute otitis media, stage 1: eustachian tube obstruction. Acute otitis media is an acute bacterial infection of the mucosal lining of the middle ear cleft (the eustachian tube, middle ear, mastoid antrum, and mastoid air cells). The most commonly encountered causative organisms include *Staphylococcus aureus*, hemolytic streptococci, *Pneumococcus*, and *Haemophilus influenzae*. These microorganisms reach the middle ear by ascending the eustachian tube from the nasopharynx, frequently following a viral upper respiratory tract infection.

Although the progression of acute otitis media has classically been divided into a series of stages, each with characteristic symptoms and otoscopic appearance, in practice, this disease usually progresses rapidly, with no clearly separated staging.

The earliest clinical sign seen in acute otitis media consists of redness and swelling in the pars flaccida. The normal luster of the tympanic membrane is lost. Initially, a mild hearing loss with a stuffy feeling in the ear or slight pain might be the only complaint. In children, this stage is usually silent.

FIGURE 3-19

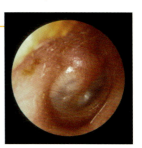

Acute otitis media, stage 2: redness. The manubrial and circumferential vessels supplying the tympanic membrane dilate, and the entire tympanic membrane eventually becomes uniformly fiery red. At this stage, there is increasing earache and hearing loss. Systemic symptoms are now usually present, including fever, nausea, vomiting, and, in children, abdominal pain or diarrhea.

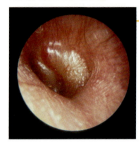

Figure 3–20

Acute otitis media, stage 3: suppuration. In severe or untreated cases, creamy white pus forms under pressure within the middle ear, and the tympanic membrane bulges outwards. The posterosuperior portion of the tympanic membrane becomes especially prominent. The bacterial infection within the middle ear can spread directly into the tympanic membrane, initially causing necrosis and rupture of the radial blood vessels. Rupture of the radial vessels appears as hemorrhagic patches in the tympanic membrane. The pain is often excruciating at this stage, and the systemic symptoms increase in severity.

At the point of rupture, prior to bursting, the drum is grayish, indicating ischemic necrosis of the fibrous middle layer. At this stage, the tympanic membrane, can be considered as the outer wall of an abscess cavity. It ulcerates on the inner surface, perforating to allow drainage of the abscess with relief of pain.

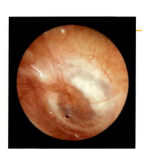

Figure 3–21

Acute otitis media, stage 4: resolution. After the tympanic membrane has ruptured, the ear becomes less painful, and otorrhea is the principal complaint. Healing of the perforation usually occurs after the infection has resolved.

Figure 3–22

Acute otitis media: resolution. A small perforation in an inflamed tympanic membrane is seen, often with a bead of pus coming from it together with pus in the external canal. Resolution occurs slowly, and the tympanic membrane will usually heal spontaneously in a few days. The tympanic membrane does not assume a fully normal appearance for approximately 6 weeks after the onset of an attack of acute otitis media.

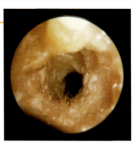

Figure 3–23

Acute mastoiditis. Today, acute mastoiditis is a relatively infrequent complication of acute suppurative otitis media. Inadequate, incomplete, or inappropriate antibiotic therapy prescribed in the treatment of acute suppurative otitis media probably suppresses the infective process just enough to prevent spontaneous rupture of the tympanic membrane ("nature's myringotomy"). The infection then continues in a relatively asymptomatic manner, and the presence of a developing coalescent mastoiditis is often hidden until it appears as a postauricular subperiosteal abscess (Figure 3–24) or as a serious intracranial complication (brain abscess or purulent meningitis).

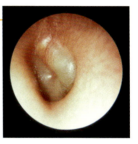

The tympanic membrane in mastoiditis is always abnormal in appearance. In untreated cases, it can be red and bulging, and the posterosuperior external canal wall will be edematous and displaced downwards by intratympanic pus. More commonly, however, the patient has been treated with antibiotics, which alter the natural course of the disease, and the tympanic membrane simply appears dull and grayish, resembling a resolving otitis media.

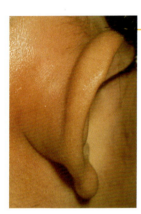

Figure 3–24

Acute mastoiditis: postauricular abscess. The symptoms can be minimal in masked mastoiditis and consist of lassitude and a low-grade fever associated with an elevated white blood cell count occurring 2 to 3 weeks after the onset of acute otitis media. There can also be tenderness of the mastoid.

The suspicion that mastoiditis has developed is based on clinical observations: a continuing low-grade fever and an abnormal tympanic membrane, or pain or swelling over the mastoid. The diagnosis is confirmed by computed tomography (CT scan).

Figure 3–25

Tympanic membrane crust. A crust is a localized accumulation of corneocytes and dried inflammatory exudate located on the surface of the tympanic membrane. Crusts vary in size, from those covering only a small area of the tympanic membrane to those covering its entire surface. Crust formation on the surface of the tympanic membrane is the result of a local infection of the tympanic membrane that occurs in those severe cases of acute otitis media where the infection within the middle ear spreads laterally into the tissues of the tympanic membrane. This localized infection produces a rapid accumulation of surface corneocytes into which a serous-like inflammatory exudate from the outer surface of the inflamed drum is absorbed.

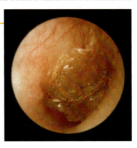

Figure 3–26

Migrating tympanic membrane crust. No treatment is necessary because over time, the crust detaches from the surface of the tympanic membrane by the normal centrifugal migration of the underlying epithelium and is then gradually carried out of the external canal on top of the normal migrating epithelium.

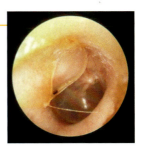

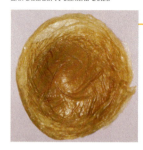

Figure 3–27

Tympanic membrane cast. A crust that has become detached from the surface of the tympanic membrane is called a "cast." The medial surface of a detached cast usually duplicates the surface contours of the underlying tympanic membrane.

Casts and crusts are usually asymptomatic. The observation of a crust on the surface of the tympanic membrane, or of a cast within the external canal, indicates that the patient has had a recent (within the previous few weeks or months) episode of severe acute suppurative otitis media.

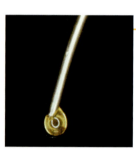

Figure 3–28

Serous otitis media: aspirated serous fluid. Serous otitis media is caused by a failure of the eustachian tube to aerate the middle ear cleft. The resulting persistent negative pressure within the middle ear appears to encourage an outpouring of a thin, sterile, golden-yellow, watery fluid from the mucoperiosteum, which lines the middle ear cleft. Eustachian tube dysfunction can result from a variety of causes, including upper respiratory tract viral infection, enlarged adenoids, allergy of the upper respiratory tract, otitic barotrauma, cleft-palate deformities, tumors of the nasopharynx, and local radiation therapy.

Serous otitis media is characterized by the presence of a nonpurulent collection of **thin, watery, clear fluid** in the middle ear cleft.

Figure 3–29

Serous otitis media. The otoscopic appearances of serous otitis media are protean and vary from an apparently normal tympanic membrane to one that is severely retracted. The color of the tympanic membrane will vary according to the color of the underlying transudate. The presence of a thin, serous effusion within the middle ear generally gives the tympanic membrane a yellowish discoloration.

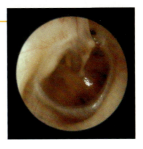

Because the fluid within the middle ear is clear and transparent, the examiner can look through the fluid and see the underlying middle ear structures.

Figure 3–30

Serous otitis media after autoinflation. Medical treatment is directed towards the restoration of normal eustachian tube function by the use of topical and/or systemic nasal decongestants combined with attempts at reinflation of the middle ear by the Valsalva maneuver (autoinflation).

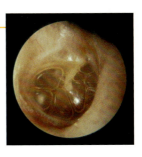

Figure 3–31

Serous otitis media: air-fluid level. In cases of incomplete eustachian tube obstruction, or following autoinflation, air bubbles (see Figure 3–30) or an air-fluid level (shown here) may be seen.

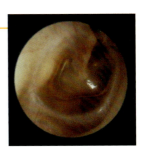

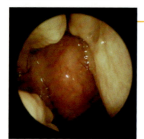

Figure 3–32

Serous otitis media secondary to nasopharyngeal carcinoma. The presence of a persistent or recurrent serous otitis media in an adult might signify the presence of an underlying carcinoma of the nasopharynx. The nasopharynx must be examined, preferably with a nasal endoscope or flexible nasopharyngoscope. If there is any doubt about the diagnosis, the nasopharynx should be examined directly under general anesthesia to rule out the presence of an underlying carcinoma.

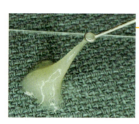

Figure 3–33

Mucoid otitis media: aspirated mucus (otitis media with effusion, secretory otitis media, glue ear). Mucoid otitis media is the most common cause of acquired conductive hearing loss in children. Mucoid otitis media is characterized by the accumulation of a thick, opalescent, tenacious mucoid effusion within the middle ear cleft. The thick mucoid effusion is the result of the normal response of the middle ear mucosa to inflammation within the middle ear.

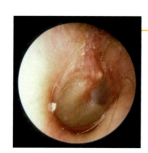

Figure 3–34

Mucoid otitis media secondary to acute otitis media. The ascent of a viral upper respiratory infection into the middle ear via the eustachian tube is the most common cause of middle ear inflammation in childhood. Antibiotic-suppressed and incompletely resolved acute suppurative otitis media might also be a significant factor in the pathogenesis of this condition in some children.

The only symptom of significance in the condition is a conductive hearing loss. Mucoid otitis media is frequently asymptomatic in children and may present only indirectly, in the form of inattention, slow language development, or poor school performance, of which it is a major cause.

FIGURE 3–35

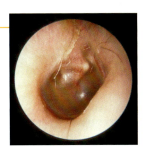

Mucoid otitis media. As in serous otitis media, the otoscopic appearances of mucoid otitis media can vary from an apparently normal tympanic membrane to one that is retracted or even slightly bulging. The radial vessels of the drum are often dilated, especially when there has been a prior episode of acute suppurative otitis media.

FIGURE 3–36

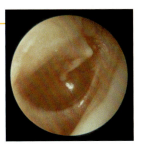

Mucoid otitis media showing discoloration of the tympanic membrane. The presence of the thick mucoid effusion within the middle ear is responsible for the dull texture and pearly gray discoloration of the tympanic membrane. **The opalescence of the effusion prevents the examiner from looking through the middle ear and, consequently, the underlying normal middle ear structures cannot be seen.** Air-fluid levels are not commonly seen in patients with mucoid otitis media.

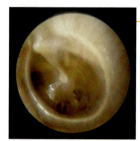

Figure 3–37

Serous otitis media prior to myringotomy. A myringotomy (small surgial incision through the tympanic membrane) is usually performed for one of three reasons: to determine if fluid is present in the middle ear, to establish drainage of the purulent contents of the middle ear in the advanced stages of acute suppurative otitis media, and to aspirate nonpurulent effusions. Currently, myringotomies are most commonly performed in the treatment of persistent serous otitis media.

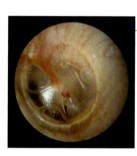

Figure 3–38

Serous otitis media immediately after myringotomy. When a myringotomy is necessary for the aspiration of fluid from a noninfected middle ear, eg, in serous or mucoid otitis media, a radial incision is preferred, because fewer of the radial tympanic blood vessels are transected. Spontaneous closure of the myringotomy incision will usually occur within 5 to 7 days after drainage from the middle ear ceases, leaving a barely perceptible scar.

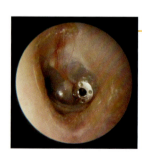

Figure 3–39

Tympanostomy tubes (ventilation tubes, grommets, pressure-equalizing tubes, artificial eustachian tubes). Many cases of conductive hearing loss caused by persistent serous or mucoid otitis media require prolonged artificial middle ear ventilation. Because most myringotomy incisions heal spontaneously within a few days, little time is left for eustachian tube function to recover, and, consequently, the middle ear effusion will tend to recur. For this reason, a ventilation tube is inserted through the myringotomy incision.

Figure 3–40

Stainless-steel ventilation tube.
The most common surgical procedure currently performed in children in North America is the insertion of an artificial eustachian tube into a myringotomy incision. The primary function of the artificial eustachian tube is to provide ventilation of the middle ear cleft by allowing the free passage of air through the tympanic membrane.

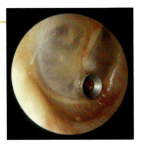

Figure 3–41

Silastic T tympanostomy tube.
Most tubes are designed with an inner flange to delay extrusion, and they often feature an outer flange to prevent the tube's falling into the middle ear (see Figure 3–39). Because the lumina of most tubes will allow water to pass from the deep external canal into the middle ear, individuals should exercise care while showering, washing their hair, or swimming to prevent water from entering the middle ear and possible subsequent infection.

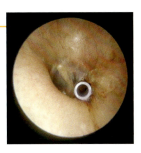

Figure 3–42

Castelli semipermeable membrane tympanostomy tube. Tubes are available in a wide range of designs, sizes, colors, and materials. The tube shown here features a gas-semipermeable membrane that prevents water from entering the middle ear.

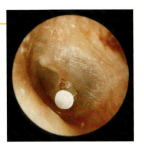

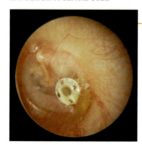

Figure 3–43

Blocked tympanostomy tube. For a tympanostomy tube to function properly, its lumen must remain patent. Premature blockage of the lumen with inspissated mucus or serous debris can lead to an early return of the middle ear effusion; replacement of the tube might then be required, although ear drops can sometimes soften the debris and clear the tube.

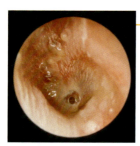

Figure 3–44

Acute otitis media with ventilation tube (AOMT). Ventilation tubes can act as drains both for middle ear effusions and for the purulent material that can develop during a subsequent episode of otitis media. This type of otitis media can be treated with a suitable topical antibiotic ear drop. The topical ear drops prescribed should be non-ototoxic.

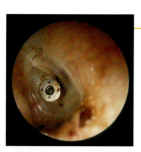

Figure 3–45

Blocked tympanostomy tube. The lumen of the stainless steel Reutter bobbin seen in this case is blocked by clotted blood, and the serous transudate has redeveloped.

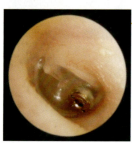

Figure 3–46

Extruding tympanostomy tube. As a result of the normal outward movement of the epithelial cells from the surface of the tympanic membrane along the ear canal, a tympanostomy tube will normally be spontaneously extruded from the tympanic membrane 6 to 12 months after insertion.

Figure 3–47

Extruding tympanostomy tube with visible collar of keratin. The underlying myringotomy incision heals in most cases. In many atelectatic ears, tympanostomy tubes are rejected quite rapidly, possibly because of atrophic changes in the tympanic membrane. This is unfortunate because the ventilation tubes are needed most in this situation.

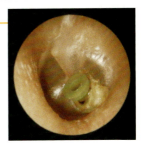

Figure 3–48

Extruding tympanostomy tube being carried laterally. After the tube has been extruded from the tympanic membrane, migration outward into the superficial portion of the external auditory canal normally occurs. The tube, often encrusted with wax, can drop out of the ear spontaneously. Otherwise, it can be removed readily.

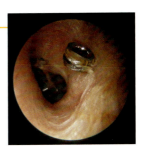

Figure 3–49

Small tube granuloma (tympanostomy tube foreign-body granuloma). In approximately 0.5% of cases, the tympanostomy tube stimulates the development of a keratin foreign-body granuloma. This is characterized by the presence of granulation tissue, with or without mucopurulent discharge, adjacent to the tympanostomy tube. A tube granuloma can be treated with a suitable non-ototoxic topical antibiotic ear drop.

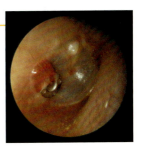

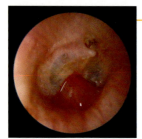

Figure 3-50

Large tube granuloma. This exuberant granulation tissue can be responsible for the development of a profuse and usually painless otorrhea that is frequently tinged with blood. A tube granuloma is treated by removal of the tube and the associated granulation tissue.

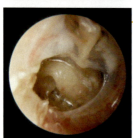

Figure 3-51

Middle ear atelectasis. Middle ear atelectasis is a severe partial or complete retraction of the tympanic membrane resulting from chronic eustachian tube dysfunction and persistent negative intratympanic pressure. After prolonged retraction, the tympanic membrane becomes thin and atrophic because of resorption of the fibrous middle layer. (Middle ear atelectasis must be differentiated from adhesive otitis media.)

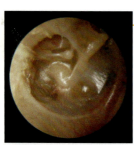

Figure 3-52

Middle ear atelectasis showing thinning of the tympanic membrane. This thinning allows the middle ear's contents to be seen more clearly than normal, and in some cases, the tympanic membrane becomes so thin that it resembles an open perforation.

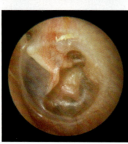

Figure 3-53

Middle ear atelectasis: retraction pocket before autoinflation. In less severe cases of middle ear atelectasis, the retraction is confined to one quadrant, whereas in advanced cases, the tympanic membrane is often firmly retracted, draped over the incus or stapes, or even draped over the promontory.

A correctly placed ventilation tube can be expected to re-aerate the middle ear, allowing the tympanic membrane to lift off the promontory.

Figure 3–54

Middle ear atelectasis: retraction pocket after autoinflation. If the patient is capable of autoinflating the middle ear, the retracted atrophic portion of the eardrum will evert. The pneumatic attachment to the otoscope can be used to confirm the diagnosis by mobilizing the thin tympanic membrane, thereby enabling the examiner to distinguish confidently a severely retracted atrophic tympanic membrane from a large central perforation.

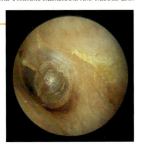

Figure 3–55

Self-cleaning retraction pocket. Prolonged negative pressure within the middle ear can "suck" a portion of the tympanic membrane medially. If the fibrous middle layer of the tympanic membrane has become thinned (atrophic), then a deeply invaginated pocket may form. This is called a "retraction pocket." Retraction pockets form most commonly in the posterosuperior quadrant of the pars tensa.

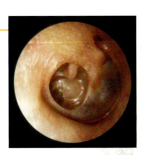

Figure 3–56

Nonself-cleaning retraction pocket. The examiner should check that the pocket is lined with normal thin and healthy epithelium. If the patient can perform a Valsalva maneuver, the pocket can be seen to balloon outwards (see Figure 3–54). Clinicians should examine retraction pockets carefully to ensure that they are self-cleansing. Those pockets that are unable to clean themselves can, over time, fill up with keratin debris and slowly enlarge until they form a cholesteatoma.

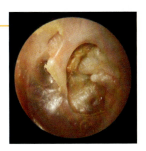

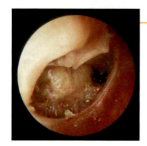

Figure 3–57

Adhesive otitis media. Adhesive otitis media is the result of a chronic process in which the tympanic membrane is retracted medially and permanently tethered to the medial wall of the middle ear by fibrous adhesions that have developed in the middle ear as the result of previous inflammatory middle ear disease. The key otoscopic feature of adhesive otitis media is severe and irreversible retraction of the tympanic membrane. The appearance of the tympanic membrane can vary from minimal scarring to overall thickening and opacity. Pneumatic otoscopy almost always discloses severe impairment or even a total absence of tympanic membrane mobility.

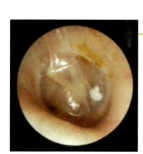

Figure 3–58

Small tympanic membrane tympanosclerosis. Tympanosclerotic plaques commonly occur in the tympanic membrane and in this location rarely produce symptoms because patches of tympanosclerosis confined to the tympanic membrane do not cause hearing loss. These chalky white plaques result from the organization of both fibrinous exudates and granulation tissue from a prior episode of severe acute otitis media.

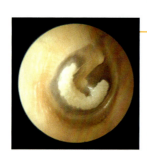

Figure 3–59

Large tympanic membrane tympanosclerosis. Tympanosclerotic plaques of the tympanic membrane are confined to the pars tensa. They range in size from tiny patches (see Figure 3–58) to those that are so large that they involving most of the fibrous middle layer of the pars tensa.

FIGURE 3–60

Middle ear tympanosclerosis. Tympanosclerosis involving the middle ear mucosa and ossicles is rare; however, when middle ear tympanosclerosis occurs, it is usually associated with a conductive hearing loss.

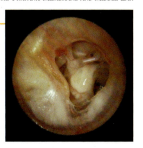

FIGURE 3–61

Small central perforation. A perforation in the pars tensa of the tympanic membrane that does not extend to involve the annulus is termed a "central perforation." Most central perforations result from a previous episode of acute otitis media and represent a failure in the healing of a tympanic membrane perforation. Central perforations can also follow severe trauma. These perforations are designated as "safe," because they are usually not associated with either cholesteatoma or the intracranial spread of infection.

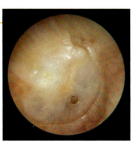

FIGURE 3–62

Medium-sized central perforation. Central perforations can vary in size from a pinhole (see Figure 3–61), through moderate (shown here), to a virtually total kidney-shaped perforation (Figure 3–63). The patient should be instructed to keep water out of the ear to avoid repeated middle ear infections.

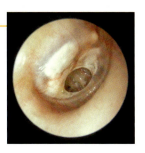

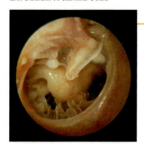

Figure 3–63

Subtotal central perforation. Often, some middle ear structures can be seen through a large subtotal perforation. The middle ear can be perfectly dry and the mucoperiosteal lining healthy in appearance.

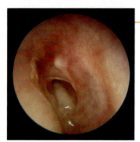

Figure 3–64

Acute otitis media with a central perforation. If the middle ear is infected, mucopurulent material will be seen through the perforation, and the mucosa is usually red and edematous. In an acutely inflamed ear, the discharge can be pulsatile. Acute otitis media with a central perforation can be treated with a suitable topical antibiotic ear drop. The topical ear drops prescribed should be non-ototoxic.

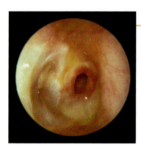

Figure 3–65

Chronic otitis media with a central perforation. In severely infected cases, mucopus, which varies in color and consistency, drains outwards through the perforation and can fill the external canal. Chronic suppurative otitis media can be treated with a suitable non-ototoxic topical antibiotic ear drop.

Figure 3–66

Healed central perforation. When a large perforation heals, the fibrous middle layer of the pars tensa is deficient, so a thin, semitransparent membrane resembling an open perforation will be seen. Gentle use of the pneumatic attachment to the otoscope will, however, demonstrate that the tympanic membrane is intact. Because the thinned segment of a healed perforation lacks the strength of a normal drum, forceful springing can result in reperforation.

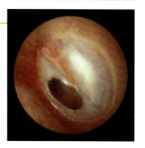

Figure 3–67

Marginal perforation. A marginal perforation involves the annulus of the pars tensa of the tympanic membrane. These perforations are considered "unsafe," because they are frequently associated with cholesteatoma. Marginal perforations involve the annulus and vary in size from a small defect to a large subtotal perforation of the tympanic membrane.

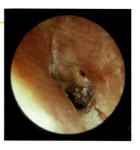

Figure 3–68

Marginal perforation with cholesteatoma. A marginal perforation located in the posterosuperior quadrant of the tympanic membrane is especially worrisome because a perforation in this area is often associated with an underlying cholesteatoma. The examiner must always have a high index of suspicion that a cholesteatoma is either present or developing within the middle ear cleft. Careful follow-up of these patients by a specialist is advisable.

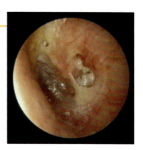

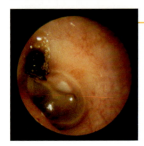

Figure 3-69

Attic crust. The presence of a crust or piece of wax obscuring the posterosuperior portion of Shrapnell's membrane must never be dismissed as trivial, because an underlying perforation, or even a cholesteatoma, is frequently present. Using the operating microscope, a clinician can usually remove the attic crust. If a small retraction pocket of an intact pars tensa is discovered, no further investigation is required; however, the patient should be followed carefully.

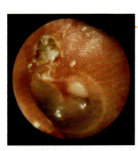

Figure 3-70

Attic cholesteatoma. When the pocket contains an obvious collection of whitish keratin squames, the presence of a cholesteatoma hidden within the middle ear is highly likely, and further investigation by CT scan is required.

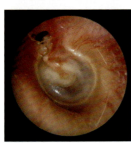

Figure 3-71

Attic perforation with cholesteatoma. An attic perforation is the hallmark of unsafe chronic suppurative otitis media. After treating overt infection with aural toilet, suction, and local antibiotic drugs, the clinician must examine the ear with an operating microscope to determine whether granulation tissue or a cholesteatoma lies within. Extensive underlying bony destruction of the incus and medial wall of the attic might have occurred "around the corner" out of view and cannot be identified through a small attic perforation. A high-resolution CT scan is mandatory.

FIGURE 3–72

Aural polyp. Most aural polyps are inflammatory in origin and occur as a result of chronic inflammation. Occasionally, a neoplasm will present as an aural polyp. Aural polyps can arise either from the external auditory canal or from the middle ear.

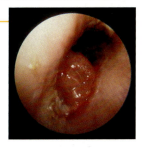

FIGURE 3–73

Attic aural polyp with cholesteatoma. Aural polyps that arise from the attic (pars flaccida of the tympanic membrane) are almost invariably associated with an underlying cholesteatoma.

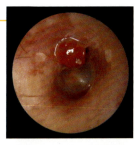

FIGURE 3–74

Cholesteatoma: keratin squame debris seen through a large tympanic membrane perforation. A cholesteatoma is a collection of keratin debris produced and enclosed by a sac of stratified squamous keratinizing epithelium located within the middle ear cleft. The keratin desquamated from the epithelium lining this pocket collects within, producing a gradually enlarging cyst. As the cyst expands, it erodes the surrounding bony walls of the middle ear and ossicles.

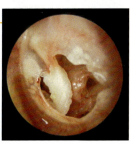

In the case shown here, keratin squame debris can be seen protruding through the large tympanic membrane perforation.

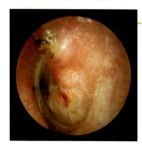

Figure 3-75

Cholesteatoma medial to the tympanic membrane. The only sign of a large cholesteatoma in the mastoid antrum or air cells is often either a few shiny white keratin squames visible through a small attic perforation or the outline of a white mass behind the tympanic membrane.

It is dangerous to overlook the presence of squamous epithelium located medial to the tympanic membrane or in the mastoid air cells because, over time, gradual bony erosion can lead to life-threatening complications such as labyrinthitis, meningitis, or brain abscess.

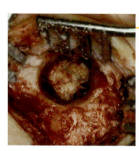

Figure 3-76

Mastoidectomy for cholesteatoma. Small cholesteatomas that can be cleaned completely by suction under the operating microscope can be managed by regular debridement and close observation. With larger pockets, in all but the elderly, the treatment of this disease is surgical and requires a mastoid exploration with either removal or exteriorization of the cholesteatoma.

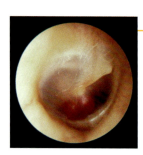

Figure 3-77

Glomus tympanicum tumor. A glomus tumor is a slowly growing, locally invasive, vascular tumor arising from the glomus bodies. A glomus tympanicum arises from glomus bodies on the medial wall of the middle ear. The earliest sign is redness behind the tympanic membrane, which is caused by the presence of this highly vascular tumor within the middle ear.

Figure 3–78

Glomus jugulare tumor. A glomus jugular arises from the glomus bodies over the jugular bulb (the floor of the middle ear). The tumor can appear as a blue or red "rising sun," seen behind the inferior portion of the tympanic membrane. The red color of the tympanic membrane often decreases if it can be lifted off the tumor by the pneumatic otoscope. In more advanced cases, the tumor can present as a red vascular polyp within the external canal that can bleed profusely on manipulation.

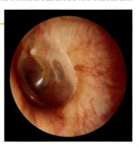

A glomus tumor will usually present with a unilateral hearing loss and an associated pulsatile roaring or rushing tinnitus.

Glomus tumors can be treated by radiotherapy, embolization of the feeding arterial blood supply, surgical extirpation, or a combination thereof.

Figure 3–79

Abnormally high jugular bulb. An abnormally high jugular bulb can also give a rising-sun appearance similar to that of a glomus jugulare tumor.

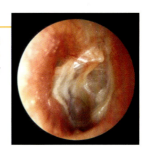

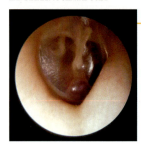

Figure 3–80

Aberrant carotid artery. An aberrant carotid artery can also give a rising-sun appearance similar to that of a glomus jugulare tumor. A jugular venogram will demonstrate the relationship of this lesion to the jugular bulb, and a carotid arteriogram will help demonstrate the vascular nature of the lesion and determine its blood supply. A CT scan can be used to delineate the extent of the tumor.

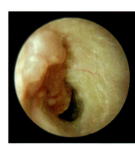

Figure 3–81

Squamous cell carcinoma of the middle ear. Squamous cell carcinoma is an uncommon malignant tumor arising from the skin of the external auditory canal or the lining of the tympanic cavity. Pain in the presence of otorrhea is the most common symptom, and chronic irritation from prolonged otorrhea appears to be a significant etiologic factor. The development of pain in any chronically infected ear should be considered a warning sign that a malignant tumor might be present. An exuberant polyp or a growth extending into the meatus, especially if it is nodular, friable, or hemorrhagic, is particularly suspect.

The earliest sign of a carcinoma is a redness (see Figure 3–77) behind the tympanic membrane, caused by the presence of this highly vascularized tumor within the middle ear.

When carcinoma is suspected, careful examination of cranial nerves seven, nine, ten, eleven, and twelve must be performed to determine whether extratympanic spread and involvement of the jugular foramen has occurred. If the tympanometer is used at its most sensitive setting, pulsatile movements transmitted from the vascular tumor to the tympanic membrane may be recorded. In all patients with unilateral pulsatile tinnitus, the possibility of an underlying vascular tumor or arteriovenous malformation should be considered.

INDEX

Aberrant carotid artery, 86
Accessory auricle, 4
Acute mastoiditis, 65
   postauricular abscess, 66
Acute otitis media, 62–65
   with central perforation, 80
   mucoid otitis media secondary to, 70
   resolution, 65
   stage 1, 62–63
   stage 2, 63
   stage 3, 64
   stage 4, 64
   suppurative, acute mastoiditis from, 65
   with ventilation tube, 74
Acute perichondritis, 12–13
Acute suppurative otitis media, acute mastoiditis from, 65
Adhesive otitis media, 78
Air pressure, traumatic tympanic membrane perforation from, 55, 57–58
Aminoglycoside ear drops, ototoxicity of, 44–45
Antibiotics, ototoxicity of, 44–45
Arteriovenous malformation, of the pinna, 23
Artificial Eustachian tubes, 72–75
Aspergillus niger, in the middle ear, 46–47
Attic aural polyp, with cholesteatoma, 83
Attic cholesteatoma, 82
Attic crust, 82
Attic perforation, with cholesteatoma, 82
Aural polyp, 83
   attic, with cholesteatoma, 83
Auricle
   accessory, 4
   squamous cell carcinoma of the, 24
Auricular cartilage, 1
   frost bite of, 10–11
      late calcification from, 11
   traumatic seroma of, 7
Auricular pseudocyst, 7
Auspitz sign, 18
Autoinflation
   refraction pocket after, 77
   refraction pocket before, 76
   serous otitis media after, 69
Automastoidectomy, from keratosis obturans, 37

Barotraumatic otitis media, 57–58
Basal cell carcinoma, 23
Bleeding, from external-canal laceration, 34
Blisters, on the tympanic membrane, 61
Blood clot
   fresh, 35
   inspissated, 35
Bullous myringitis, 61
   showing blebs filled with serosanguineous fluid, 61

Canal stenosis, 49
Candida albicans, 17, 46–47
Capillary hemangioma, 22
Carcinoma
   basal cell, 23
   serous otitis media secondary to nasocarcinoma, 70
   squamous cell
      of the auricle, 24
      of external auditory canal, 53
      keratoacanthoma and, 22
      of the middle ear, 86–87
      solar keratosis and, 21
   verrucous, 24
Carotid artery, aberrant, 86
Cast, tympanic membrane, 67–68
Castelli semipermeable membrane tympanostomy tube, 73
Cauliflower ear, 9
Cerumen
   accumulation, 31
   colors of, 31
   dry, 32
   normal, 30
   "oriental," 32
   "true" color of, 31
   veil of, 31
   wet, 32
Cerumenolytics
   effective, 32
   ineffective, 33
Ceruminous glands, 30
"Chocolate eardrum," 59
Cholesteatoma

attic, 82
attic aural polyp with, 83
attic perforation with, 82
defined, 83
keratin squame debris through a large tympanic membrane perforation, 83
mastoidectomy for, 84
medial to the tympanic membrane, 84
perforation marginal with, 81
Chondrodermatitis nodularis helicus chronica, 20
Chorda tympani, 29
Chronic infective dermatitis, 17, 25
Chronic otitis media, with central perforation, 80
Cold water, exostoses and, 40
Congenital malformations, of the pinna, 24–25
Contact dermatitis
   of external ear, 14–15
   metal, of the lobule, 15
   from neomycin, 48
Cotton swab abuse, 33
   chronic otitis externa from, 48
   external-canal hematoma from, 33–34
Creased lobule, 13
Crust
   attic, 82
   tympanic membrane, 67–68
Cutaneous horn, 21
Cystic chondromalacia, idiopathic, 7
Cysts
   epidermal, 16–17
   epidermal inclusion, 35
   preauricular, 5

Darwin's tubercle, 1
Dermatitis
   chronic infective, 17, 25
   contact
      of external ear, 14–15
      metal of the lobule, 15
      from neomycin, 48
   neurodermatitis, 17
   solar of the pinna, 10

Ear mold pressure ulceration, 10
Earring hole
   elongated, 14

89

infected, 14
Ear wax. *See* Cerumen
Effusion, otitis media with, 70
Epidermal cysts, 16
  drainage of infected, 17
  infected, 17
  post-traumatic inclusion, 16
  showing cheesy debris, 16
Epidermal inclusion cyst, 35
Epithelial migration, normal, 27–28, 30
Eustachian tube, artificial, 72–75
Exostoses
  arising from tympanic bone, 40
  blocking the canal, 41
  cold water and, 40
  CT scan of, 40
  large solitary, 40
  multiple, 41
  small solitary, 40
External auditory canal, 26
  bony portion of, 27
  cartilaginous, 26
  laceration of, 34
  normal epithelial migration, 27–28, 30
  self-cleansing properties of, 27–28
  squamous cell carcinoma of, 53
  stenosis of
    moderate, 49
    severe, 49
  transverse wrinkles of the deep canal, 30
  tympanic bone, 26
  tympanic membrane, 28–29
External-canal hematoma
  large, 34
  small, 33

False fundus, 50
Foreign-body
  cockroach, 39
  foam rubber, 39
  large pebble, 39
  plastic bead, 38
  Schuknecht remover, 39
  in tympanostomy tube, 75
Frostbite, of the pinna, 10–11
Fundus, false, 50
Fungal infection
  in epidermal cysts, 17
  in otitis externa, 46–47

Furuncle, 42

Glomus jugulare tumor, 85
Glomus tympanicum tumor, 84
Glue ear, 70
Gouty tophus, 19
Granular myringitis, 62
Granuloma
  keratin foreign-body, 35
  large tube, 76
  small tube, 75
  tympanostomy tube foreign-body, 75
Grommets, 72

Haemophilus influenza, 62
Hairy pinna, 6
Hairy tragus, 6
Hearing aid, ear mold pressure ulceration from, 10
Hearing loss
  in bullous myringitis, 61
  veil of cerumen, 31
Hemangioma, capillary, 22
Hematoma
  external-canal
    large, 34
    small, 33
  subperichonrial
    large, 8
    small, 9
Hemotympanum, 59
  aspirate from, 59
  "chocolate eardrum," 59
Herpes zoster
  of the pinna
    early, 11
    late, 11
  of the tympanic membrane, 12
Herpes zoster oticus, 52–53
Hypertrichosis lanuginosa acquisita, 7
Hypertrophic scars, 15

Idiopathic cystic chondromalacia, 7
Impetigo, of the pinna, 12
Irradiation osteitis, 38

Jugular bulb
  aberrant carotid artery, 86
  abnormally high, 85
  glomus jugulare tumor, 85

Keloids, 15
Keratin debris, 36. *See also* Cholesteatoma

chronic otitis externa with, 47
Keratin foreign-body granuloma, 35
Keratin patches
  demonstrated by osmium staining, 30
  on normal tympanic membrane, 29
Keratoacanthoma, 22
Keratosis
  neglect, 18
  seborrheic, 18
  solar, 21
Keratosis obturans, 36
  automastoidectomy, 37
  debris from, 36
  treatment guidelines, 37
  widened deep canal, 36

Laceration of external-canal, 34
Lentigo, solar, 20
Lobule
  creased, 13
  elongated earring hole, 14
  metal contact dermatitis of, 15
  split, 14

Malignant otitis externa, 51–52
Mastoidectomy, for cholesteatoma, 84
Mastoiditis, acute, 65
  postauricular abscess, 66
Meatal atresia
  complete, 2
  partial, 2
Microtia, 3
Middle ear
  barotrauma, 57
    showing serous exudate, 58
  squamous cell carcinoma of the, 86–87
  tympanosclerosis, 79
Middle ear atelectasis, 76
  refraction pocket after autoinflation, 77
  refraction pocket before autoinflation, 76
  showing thinning of the tympanic membrane, 76
Middle ear tympanosclerosis, 79
Migration, normal epithelial, 27–28, 30
Milia, 16
Mucoid otitis media, 70–71
  aspirated mucus of, 70

secondary to acute otitis media, 70
Mycoplasma pneumoniae, 61
Myringitis
  bullous, 61
    showing blebs filled with serosanguineous fluid, 61
  granular, 62
Myringitis bullosa, 61
Myringotomy
  serous otitis media immediately after, 72
  serous otitis media prior to, 72
  tympanostomy tubes and, 72

Nasocarcinoma, serous otitis media secondary to, 70
Necrotizing otitis externa, 51–52
Neglect keratosis, 18
Neomycin, contact dermatitis from, 48
Neurodermatitis, 17
Nevus, pigmented, 21
Normal epithelial migration, of external auditory canal, 27–28, 30

Obturans, keratosis, 36–37
Osteitis
  benign, of the external auditory canal, 37–38
  irradiation, 38
Osteoma, of the external auditory canal, 41
Otitis externa, 42–51
  acute
    allergic, 48
    circumscribed, 42
    early diffuse, 43
    severe diffuse, 43
  aspergillus, 46
    acute, 46
    severe, 46
    severe acute, 47
  chronic
    candidal, 47
    from chronic cotton bud use, 48
    with keratin debris, 47
    with purulent exudates, 48
    fungal infection, 46–47
  malignant, 51–52
  necrotizing, 51–52
  Pope Otowick for, 44
  treatment, 43–45

Otitis media
  acute, 62–65
    with central perforation, 80
    mucoid otitis media secondary to, 70
    resolution, 65
    stage 1, 62–63
    stage 2, 63
    stage 3, 64
    stage 4, 64
    suppurative, acute mastoiditis from, 65
    with ventilation tube, 74
  adhesive, 78
  chronic, with central perforation, 80
  with effusion, 70
  mucoid, 70–71
    aspirated mucus of, 70
    secondary to acute otitis media, 70
  secretory, 70
  serous, 68–70, 72
    after autoinflation, 69
    air-fluid level, 69
    immediately after myringotomy, 72
    prior to myringotomy, 72
    secondary to nasocarcinoma, 70
    signs and symptoms of, 68
    showing discoloration of the tympanic membrane, 71
Otomycosis, 46
Ototopical antibiotics, ototoxicity of, 44–45
Ototoxicity, 44–45
Outstanding ears
  lateral view, 4
  posterior view, 3

Pars flaccida, 29
Pars tensa, 28
Peau d'orange, 43
Perforation
  attic, with cholesteatoma, 82
  healed central, 81
  marginal, 81
  marginal with cholesteatoma, 81
  medium-sized central, 79
  small central, 79
  subtotal central, 80
  traumatic, 55–57
    direct, 57
    healing, 56

healing direct, 57
mechanism of, 55
Perichondritis
  acute, 12–13
  relapsing, 13
Physical trauma
  cauliflower ear from, 9
  external-canal hematoma from, 33–34
  traumatic tympanic membrane perforation from, 55, 57
Pigmented nevus, 21
Pinna
  auricular cartilage of, 1
  congenital malformations of the, 24–25
  hairy, 6
  meatal atresia, 2
  microtia, 3
  normal, 1
Polyp, aural, 83
Pope Otowick
  inserted in an occluded ear canal, 44
  for otitis externa, 44
Postauricular abscess, acute mastoiditis, 66
Preauricular cyst, 5
Preauricular pit, 5
Preauricular sinus, infected, 5–6
Preauricular tag, 4
Pressure-equalizing tubes, 72–75
Proteus, 13
Pseudomonas aeruginosa, 13, 43, 51
Psoriasis, 18
  of the external canal, 19

Ramsey hunt syndrome, 52–53
Refraction pocket
  after autoinflation, 77
  before autoinflation, 76
  nonself-cleaning, 77
  self-cleaning, 77
Relapsing perichondritis, 13

Schuknecht foreign-body remover, 39
Seborrheic keratosis, 18
Secretory otitis media, 70
Serous otitis media, 68–70, 72
  after autoinflation, 69
  air-fluid level, 69
  immediately after myringotomy, 72
  prior to myringotomy, 72

secondary to naso-carcinoma, 70
signs and symptoms of, 68
Shingles
of the pinna, 11
of tympanic membrane, 12
Shrapnell's membrane, 29, 82
Silastic T tympanostomy tubes, 73
Solar dermatitis, of the pinna, 10
Solar keratosis, 21
Solar lentigo, 20
Squamous cell carcinoma
of the auricle, 24
of external auditory canal, 53
keratoacanthoma and, 22
of the middle ear, 86–87
solar keratosis and, 21
Staphylococcus aureus, 12, 17, 62
Strawberry birthmark, 22
Streptococcus, 17
group beta-hemolytic, 13
Streptococcus pyogenes, 12
Subperichonrial hematoma
large, 8
postdrainage, 9
small, 9
Sunburn
chondrodermatitis nodularis helicus chronica and, 20
keratoacanthoma, 22
of the pinna, 10
solar keratosis and, 21
solar lentigo and, 20
Swimmer's ear, 43

Temporal bone fracture, 60
Temporomandibular perforation, ototoxicity precautions with, 45
Tophus, gouty, 19
Tragus, hairy, 6

Transverse wrinkles of the deep canal, 30
Trauma
barotrauma, 55, 57–58
physical
cauliflower ear from, 9
external-canal hematoma from, 33–34
traumatic tympanic membrane perforation from, 55, 57
Traumatic perforation, 55–57
direct, 57
healing, 56
healing direct, 57
mechanism of, 55
Traumatic seroma, 7
aspirate from, 8
Tumor
glomus jugulare, 85
glomus tympanicum, 84
osteoma of the external auditory canal, 41
Tympanic bone, 26
exostoses arising from, 40
Tympanic membrane
apparent shape of, 55
cholesteatoma medial to the, 84
congenital epidermal inclusion cyst of, 55
in herpes zoster oticus, 53
normal, 28, 54
keratin patches, 29
layers of, 28
pars flaccida, 29
pars tensa, 28
vascular strip, 29
shingles of, 12
spontaneous rupture of, 65
traumatic perforation, 55–57. *See also* Perforation
direct, 57
healing, 56
healing direct, 57

mechanism of, 55
true shape of, 55
Tympanic membrane crust, 67–68
migrating, 67
Tympanic membrane tympanosclerosis
large, 78
small, 78
Tympanicum tumor, glomus, 84
Tympanosclerosis, tympanic membrane, 78
Tympanosclerotic plaques, 78
Tympanostomy tubes, 72–75. *See also* Ventilation tube
blocked, 74
Castelli semipermeable membrane, 73
extruding, 74
carried laterally, 75
with visible collar of keratin, 75
foreign-body granuloma, 75
Silastic T, 73
stainless-steel ventilation tubes, 73

Ulceration, from hearing aid ear mold, 10
Uric acid crystals, 19

Valsalva maneuver, 69
Varicella zoster, 11–12
Vascular strip, of tympanic membrane, 29
Veil of cerumen, 31
Ventilation tube, 72–75. *See also* Tympanostomy tubes
acute otitis media with, 74
stainless-steel, 73
Verruca vulgaris, 21
Verrucous carcinoma, 24

Wart, of external ear, 21
Winkler's nodule, 20